Patents Book Series
"Topics in Anti-Cancer Research"

(Volume 8)

Edited by

Atta-ur-Rahman, *FRS*
Honorary Life Fellow, Kings College, University of Cambridge, Cambridge, UK

&

Khurshid Zaman
Bentham Science Publishers, USA

Topics in Anti-Cancer Research

Volume # 8

Editors: Atta-ur-Rahman, *FRS* and Khurshid Zaman

ISSN (Print): 2468-5860

ISSN (Online): 2213-3585

ISBN (Online): 978-981-14-0438-2

ISBN (Print): 978-981-14-0437-5

©2019, Bentham Books imprint.

Published by Bentham Science Publishers – Sharjah, UAE. All Rights Reserved.

need for a court order if at any point you breach any terms of this License Agreement. In no event will any delay or failure by Bentham Science Publishers in enforcing your compliance with this License Agreement constitute a waiver of any of its rights.

3. You acknowledge that you have read this License Agreement, and agree to be bound by its terms and conditions. To the extent that any other terms and conditions presented on any website of Bentham Science Publishers conflict with, or are inconsistent with, the terms and conditions set out in this License Agreement, you acknowledge that the terms and conditions set out in this License Agreement shall prevail.

Bentham Science Publishers Pte. Ltd.
80 Robinson Road #02-00
Singapore 068898
Singapore
Email: subscriptions@benthamscience.net

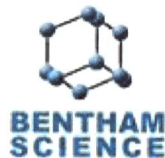

BENTHAM SCIENCE

CONTENTS

FOREWORD

Topics in Anti-Cancer Research covers new developments in the field of cancer. Novel drugs as anticancer agents include natural and synthetic phenazines and other anti-cancer compounds. It also encompasses the role of estrogen as endocrine disruptors and strategies targeting cancer stem cells for the treatment of different types of cancers including myeloma and renal cell cancer.

The topics covered in the eighth volume of this series are as follows:

• Novel Drugs for Multiple Myeloma
• Synthetic Estrogens are Endocrine Disruptors via Inhibition of AF1 Domain of ERs
• Recent Progress of Phenazines as Anticancer Agents
• Cancer Stem Cell Targeting for Anticancer Therapy: Strategies and Challenges

Robak has presented novel drugs as anticancer agents for the treatment of different types of cancers, including myeloma, along with their mechanisms of action.

The chapter by Suba deals with recent advances in the development of new drugs, which can lead to more effective therapies for cancer patients. Recent patent literature has been discussed regarding the role of estrogen as an endocrine disruptor through the inhibition of AF1 Domain of liganded and unliganded Estrogen Receptors (ERs).

Hussain *et al.* have reviewed natural and potent synthetic phenazines and which show potent anticancer activities.

Novel strategies and challenges for targeting cancer stem cells, and recent patents in the area of cancer stem cells targeting have been presented in the next chapter by Das *et al.*

The diversity of researches and topics published in this Book Series will be valuable to our cancer researchers, clinicians, cancer professional's aiming to develop novel anti-cancer targets and patents for the treatment of varied cancers.

We are thankful to the authors for their contributions and to the reviewers for their valuable comments for improving the quality of chapters. We extend our thanks to Mr. Mahmood Alam, Mrs. Rafia Rehan and other colleagues for their cooperation in the completion of this volume.

Atta-ur-Rahman, *FRS*
International Center for Chemical and Biological Sciences
University of Karachi
Karachi 75270
Pakistan

Khurshid Zaman
Honorary Editor
Bentham Science Publishers

INTRODUCTION

Topics in Anti-Cancer Research covers new developments in the field of cancer. Novel drugs as anticancer agents include natural and synthetic phenazines and other anti-cancer compounds. It also encompasses the role of estrogen as endocrine disruptors and strategies targeting cancer stem cells for the treatment of different types of cancers, including myeloma and renal cell cancer.

The diversity of researches and topics published in this Book Series will be valuable to cancer researchers, clinicians, and cancer professionals aiming to develop novel anti-cancer targets for the treatment of various cancers.

The topics covered in the eighth volume of this series are as follows:

- Novel Drugs for Multiple Myeloma
- Synthetic Estrogens are Endocrine Disruptors via Inhibition of AF1 Domain of ERs
- Recent Progress of Phenazines as Anticancer Agents
- Cancer Stem Cell Targeting for Anticancer Therapy: Strategies and Challenges

List of Contributors

Abbas, Ghulam Department of Biological Sciences and Chemistry, University of Nizwa, Birkat Al-Mauz, P.O.Box 33, Nizwa 616, Oman
Email: abbashej@unizwa.edu.om

Chakraborty, Tapash Girijananda Chowdhury Institute of Pharmaceutical Science, Hatkhowapara, Azara, Guwahati, Assam, 781017, India
Email: tapash.mpharm@gmail.com

Das, Malay K. Department of Pharmaceutical Sciences, Dibrugarh University, Dibrugarh, Assam, 786004, India
Email: mkdps@dibru.ac.in

Das, Sanjoy Department of Pharmaceutical Sciences, Dibrugarh University, Dibrugarh, Assam, 786004, India
Email: sanjoyeyeconic@gmail.com

Green, Ivan R. Department of Chemistry and Polymer Science, University of Stellenbosch, Private Bag X1, Matieland, Stellenbosch 7600, South Africa
Email: irg@sun.ac.za

Hussain, Hidayat Department of Bioorganic Chemistry, Leibniz Institute of Plant Biochemistry, Weinberg 3, D-06120 Halle (Salle), Germany
Email: hussainchem3@gmail.com

Khan, Amjad Boyle & Hooke Oxford, Hampden House, Oxford, Oxfordshire, OX44 7RW, UK
Email: amjadkhan2002@hotmail.com

Khattak, Khanzadi F. Department of Chemistry, Women University, Swabi, Swabi 23430, Pakistan
Email: khattakkf@yahoo.com

Rehman, Najeeb Ur Natural and Medical Sciences Research Center, University of Nizwa, PC 616, Nizwa, Oman
Email: najeeb@unizwa.edu.om

Robak, Pawel Department of Experimental Hematology, Medical University of Lodz Copernicus Memorial Hospital, Ul. Ciolkowskiego 2, 93-510 Lodz, Poland
Email: robakpawel@op.pl

Robak, Tadeusz Department of Hematology, Medical University of Lodz Copernicus Memorial Hospital, Ul. Ciolkowskiego 2, 93-510 Lodz, Poland
Email: robaktad@csk.umed.lodz.pl

Suba, Zsuzsanna National Institute of Oncology, Department of Molecular Pathology: H-1122, Ráth György Str. 7-9, Budapest, Hungary
Email: subazdr@gmail.com

CHAPTER 1

Novel Drugs for Multiple Myeloma

Pawel Robak and **Tadeusz Robak**[*]

Department of Hematology Medical University of Lodz, Copernicus Memorial Hospital Ul. Ciolkowskiego 2, Lodz 93-510, Poland

Abstract: Multiple Myeloma (MM) is a complex disease considered incurable in the majority of patients; however, several new treatments have been developed over the last decade, including third generation immunomodulatory drugs (pomalidomide), second generation proteasome inhibitors (carfilzomib and ixazomib), a histone deacetylase inhibitor (panobinostat) and monoclonal antibodies (elotuzumab and daratumumab). In addition, some new agents with unique mechanisms of action are in the process of development. Of these, isatuximab, oprozomib, filanesib (ARRY-520), dinaciclib, venetoclax, selinexor, melflufen and LGH-447 are the most promising, demonstrating preclinical single-agent activity against MM. In this chapter, we present the current status of newer and investigational anti-myeloma agents, and outline future directions for clinical use. We also summarize recent developments in the treatment of MM patients, obtained through a thorough literature review of all WO, EP and US patents filed in 2010-2018, using PubMed and http://ep.espacenet.com/ as sources. The development of novel drugs will hopefully lead to therapies with more potent effects.

Keywords: Afuresertib, bortezomib, citarinostat, daratumumab, elotuzumab, filanesib, ixazomib, isatuximab, lenalidomide, melflufen, nivolumab, oprozomib, panobinostat, pembrolizumab, pomalidomide, ricolinostat, selinexor, trametinib, venetoclax, vorinostat.

1. INTRODUCTION

Multiple Myeloma (MM) is characterized by the malignant proliferation of plasma cells, resulting in bone lesions, hypercalcemia, infections, anemia and production of monoclonal immunoglobulin [1]. It is the second most common adult hematologic malignancy, accounting for 1.3% of all malignancies and 15% of hematological neoplasms with an annual incidence of 4.5 to six cases per 100 000 people [2]. Approximately 86 000 new cases of MM occur annually worldwide [3]. In the United States, it was estimated that 30 280 new cases and 12

---

[*] **Corresponding author Tadeusz Robak:** Department of Hematology Medical University of Lodz Copernicus Memorial Hospital Ul. Ciolkowskiego 2, Lodz 93-510, Poland; Tel: +48 42 689-51-91; Fax: + 48 42 689-51-92; E-mail: robaktad@csk.umed.lodz.pl

Atta-ur-Rahman and Khurshid Zaman (Eds.)

590 attributable deaths occurred in 2017 [4], and its incidence has increased over the last decade, bringing with it considerable clinical, social and economic impact [5]. The median age at diagnosis is believed to be 72 years, with a mortality of 4.1/100 000/year [6].

Recent ESMO guidelines specify that a diagnosis of MM requires the presence of ≥ 10% clonal bone marrow plasma cells or biopsy-proven bony or extramedullary plasmacytoma, together with the occurrence of at least one of the following myeloma-defining events: hypercalcaemia, anaemia, bone lesions, ≥ 60% clonal Bone Marrow (BM) plasma cells or serum-free light chain ratio ≥ 100 [7]. The disease progresses from a premalignant stage called Monoclonal Gammopathy of Undetermined Significance (MGUS). MGUS is defined as a plasma cell-proliferative disorder characterized by plasma cell content of less than 10% in the BM, M-protein in serum < 30g/L, with no end organ damage and no evidence of other B-cell lymphoproliferative disorder [8]. MGUS is a common disorder in older people, accounting for 3.2% of Caucasian individuals aged over 50 years [9] and 5.3% of those aged 70 years or more. This disorder precedes the development of MM with a rate of MM transformation of 1% per year [10 - 12]. Symptomatic MM is characterized by neoplastic proliferation of a single clone of plasma cells producing M-protein, inducing end-organ damage, including bone lesions, anemia, renal insufficiency, and hypercalcemia (CRAB symptoms) [7, 8, 13]. MM remains an incurable disease with a median Overall Survival (OS) of six to 10 years depending on the age at diagnosis [6, 7].

2. PATHOGENESIS OF MULTIPLE MYELOMA

Multiple Myeloma (MM) develops from an accumulation of terminally-differentiated monoclonal plasma cells in the Bone Marrow (BM). MM tumor cells originate in the BM, but they are able to migrate into the peripheral blood and other tissues. MM is a multifocal disease characterized by spatial genomic heterogeneity, with several genetically-distinct malignant sub-clones [14]. Both the interaction between MM cells and host factors, and the BM microenvironment itself, play important roles in the molecular evolution of the disease and the generation of treatment-resistant cells; they also influence disease progression, with the possible development of relapsed or refractory MM [15]. The MM BM microenvironment is composed of osteoblasts, osteoclasts, BM stromal cells, an immunosuppressive milieu of cytokines, Myeloid-Derived Suppressor Cells (MDSC) and regulatory T cells. Interactions with the adhesion molecules on the surface of MM cells and the ECM components of the BM allow malignant plasma cells to disseminate throughout the BM microenvironment, during which, they receive multiple signals that maintain their survival and influence drug-induced apoptosis [16, 17]. MM plasma cells are typically found in the BM, where their growth, survival and potential drug resistance are fostered by the cellular and extracellular components of the microenvironment [18]. In this environment, MM cells adhere to BM cells with the aid of the VLA-4/ VCAM-1 integrin system [19].

The activation of the nuclear factor κB (NF-κB) family of transcription factors is typically dysregulated in MM cells; this results in greater stimulation of the cells due to the overexpression of several tumor-promoting cytokines, including Tumor Necrosis Factor (TNF), IL-1, IL-6 and BAFF [20]. This signaling can also stimulate the expression of pro-survival factors, including cFLIP, cIAP2, Bcl-xL and Bcl-2, which stimulate the growth of MM cells and protect them from the action of apoptosis-inducing chemotherapeutic agents. NF-κB signaling has also been implicated in the elevated expression of adhesion molecules such as ICAM1, which are produced by tumor cells in a NF-κB-dependent fashion. Elevated secretion of cytokines, mainly Vascular Endothelial Growth Factor (VEGF) and Fibroblast Growth Factor-2 (FGF-2) results in increased angiogenesis in the BM [21], accompanied by elevated interleukin-6 (IL-6) secretion by BM endothelial cells; thus hastening MM progression and weakening survival [22, 23].

Osteolysis is commonly observed in MM due to the activation of osteoclast progenitors, the initiation of osteoclastic bone resorption and the suppression of osteoblasts. This complex process is induced by the interaction between MM cells and the bone microenvironment via several intercellular signaling cascades, the key ones being RANK/RANKL/OPG, Notch and Wnt. Osteocytes play an important role in osteolysis through the production and secretion of various agents including Receptor Activator of NF-κB Ligand (RANKL), sclerostin and Dickkopf-1 (DKK-1) [24]. However, neoplastic plasma cells alter the BM microenvironment by stimulating the apoptosis of osteocytes, thus creating a premetastatic niche for further expansion of MM cells [25]. Osteoclast formation in the BM is stimulated by the adherence of MM cells via the action of the osteoclastogenic Vascular Cell Adhesion Molecule 1 (VCAM-1) and α4β1 integrin; together with RANKL, these factors are known to induce osteolysis [26]. These osteoclast-activation and bone reabsorption activities are also supported by the Interleukin- (IL-1β) and TNF-β produced by neoplastic plasma cells [27].

Cases of MM are typified by an upregulation of proteasome activity, and hence a disruption in the balance between the synthesis and degradation of proteins in the neoplastic plasma cells. As a result, excessive degradation occurs of the tumor suppressor p53 and the inhibitor of NF-κB in the Ubiquitin-Proteasome (UPS) pathway, leading to abnormalities in key cellular processes such as regulation of cell cycle progression, apoptosis, antigen presentation and transcription [28].

3. NOVEL DRUGS FOR MULTIPLE MYELOMA

In recent years, several new drugs with different mechanisms of action have transformed our approach to the treatment of patients with relapsed/refractory MM [29]. These include third-generation Immunomodulatory Drugs (IMiDs) (pomalidomide), second generation Proteasome Inhibitors (PIs) (carfilzomib and ixazomib), a histone deacetylase inhibitor (panobinostat) and monoclonal antibodies (mAbs) (elotuzumab and daratumumab). Schematic presentation of newer drugs for MM and their targets is displayed in Fig. (**1**).

Recently, the US Food and Drug Administration (FDA) and European Medicines Agency (EMA) have approved pomalidomide, carfilzomib, panobinostat, elotuzumab, ixazomib and daratumumab for the treatment of patients with refractory/relapsed MM.

4. PROTEASOME INHIBITORS

Three proteasome inhibitors (bortezomib, carfilzomib and ixazomib) were currently approved for the treatment of MM and several new drugs from this group are undergoing clinical trials (Fig. **2**). Proteasome Inhibitors (PIs) induce the Unfolded Protein Response (UPR) and, ultimately, cell apoptosis via proteasomal inhibition. The UPR mechanism is relatively more sensitive to PIs in MM cells, resulting in the synthesis of higher levels of monoclonal proteins. PIs induce cell death through various mechanisms, including the inhibition of NF-κB activity, activation of p53, accumulation of misfolded proteins, activation of c-Jun N-terminal kinase and stabilization of cell cycle inhibitors [30 - 32]. These drugs may prevent NF-κB dependent upregulation of the FA/BRCA DNA repair pathway and increase the cytotoxic effect of alkylating drugs [33]. Several novel PIs with improved pharmacodynamic or pharmacokinetic properties, such as marizomib, delanzomib or oprozomib, are currently under investigation in clinical trials [34].

4.1. Bortezomib

Bortezomib (Velcade®, Millennium/Takeda, Janssen) is a first-in-class selective, reversible inhibitor of the 26S proteasome which plays a role in the degradation of many intracellular proteins [35 - 37]. Bortezomib exerts its antiproliferative and antitumor activity by inhibiting the proteasomal degradation of several regulatory ubiquitinated proteins; however, it demonstrates high proteasomal selectivity and does not inhibit other proteases [38, 39]. It exerts substantial anti-myeloma activity in previously-untreated and relapsed/refractory MM patients either when used as a single drug or in combination with other anti-cancer agents. Several clinical trials have found it to possess clinical activity in newly-diagnosed and relapsed/refractory MM patients, as well as in maintenance therapy [40].

Bortezomib was the first proteasome inhibitor approved by the FDA fast-track route in 2003 for the treatment of relapsed and/or refractory MM patients progressing after two prior therapies [41, 42]. In 2008, the FDA approved injected bortezomib for the treatment of previously-untreated MM. In 2012, subcutaneous administration of bortezomib was approved by the FDA and EMA for all approved indications. In 2014, the FDA approved bortezomib for the retreatment of adult patients with MM whose disease had previously responded to bortezomib therapy but had relapsed at least six months after completion [43].

Although bortezomib can be administered both intravenously and subcutaneously [44], the subcutaneous route is now recommended based on the results of the large randomized Phase III trial (MMY-3021 trial) including 222 relapsed MM patients [44]. This non-inferiority trial found that subcutaneous bortezomib induced similar Overall Response (OR) rate, time to progression, and one-year Overall Survival (OS) scores as intravenous administration. In addition, subcutaneous administration was found to be associated with greater tolerability and lower peripheral neuropathy than intravenous administration. Subcutaneous bortezomib is also more convenient for patients, and this method of administration is now recommended. Importantly, renal insufficiency does not influence the safety and efficacy of bortezomib [45], and impairments in hepatic function do not significantly influence its pharmacodynamic properties [46].

In the last three years, several generic equivalents of Velcade have become available. In 2015, the European Commission granted marketing authorisation for Bortezomib Accord (Accord Healthcare Ltd.), and in 2016, the EMA approved generic Bortezomib Hospira and Bortezomib Sun [SUN Pharmaceutical Industries B.V.)]. Generic bortezomib has a lower price and is more widely used, even in lower-income countries [47].

Bortezomib is highly effective in previously untreated MM patients, including high-risk patient subgroups. The drug is also effective in older patients with comorbidities, renal insufficiency and poor-risk cytogenetics including t(4;14) translocation or del(17p) [48, 49]. Based on the results of the current Phase 3 trials, three-drug combinations including bortezomib and dexamethasone have become the standard induction regimens in previously-untreated patients prior to Autologous Stem Cell Transplantation (ASCT) [7, 50, 51]. In certain circumstances, bortezomib - dexamethasone can be effective in older patients who may be unsuitable for ASCT. Bortezomib can also be combined with bendamustine - doxorubicin or bendamustine - dexamethasone in previously-untreated and relapsed/refractory MM patients [52, 53]. Consolidation and maintenance therapy with bortezomib following Autologous Stem Cell Transplantation (ASCT) is associated with increased Progression Free Survival (PFS) and an overall improvement in OS, especially in patients with the high-risk disease [54]. A recent study indicates that bortezomib consolidation therapy is effective in delaying disease progression and improving the quality of responses in newly-diagnosed patients following ASCT, regardless of prior bortezomib exposure, and that it is generally well tolerated [55, 56].

4.2. Carfilzomib

Carfilzomib (Kyprolis, Onyx, Amgen) is a new-generation irreversible proteasome inhibitor with significant activity in relapsed or refractory MM, even in patients pretreated with bortezomib or immunomodulatory drugs. Carfilzomib has greater activity and was found to induce longer PFS than bortezomib in patients with relapsed MM. Carfilzomib was approved by the FDA in 2012 for the treatment of relapsed and refractory MM on the basis of the PX-171-003-A1 Phase 2 Study of carfilzomib in relapsed and refractory MM [57]. Subsequently, its high activity in MM patients has been confirmed in two Phase 3 trials: the ASPIRE Phase 3 study compared carfilzomib, lenalidomide and dexamethasone with lenalidomide and dexamethasone in patients with relapsed MM [58] and the ENDEAVOR Phase 3 study compared carfilzomib and dexamethasone with bortezomib and dexamethasone in relapsed MM patients [59]. Both the trials indicated that the carfilzomib combinations were more effective than those used in the control arms. In the EMN011 trial, carfilzomib was combined with pomalidomide and dexamethasone (KPD) in MM patients refractory to bortezomib and lenalidomide [60]. All the patients received four cycles of KPD; however, those who had not previously received ASCT received high dose melphalan (200mg/m^2) before ASCT, followed by consolidation with four additional cycles of KPD and pomalidomide - dexamethasone maintenance until progression. An 87% OR rate was observed, including 31% CR. At a median follow-up of 16.3 months, median PFS was 18 months

4.3. Ixazomib

Ixazomib (MLN9708; Ninlaro, Millennium/Takeda Oncology) is an oral proteasome inhibitor with high therapeutic activity in MM [61]. It was selected from boron-containing proteasome inhibitors based on a physicochemical profile distinct from bortezomib (Fig. **1**) [62]. The drug can be administered intravenously and orally. Ixazomib combined with lenalidomide and dexamethasone offered improved PFS and duration of response in patients with relapsed and/or relapsed/refractory MM in comparison with those treated with lenalidomide and dexamethasone alone [63].

Based on the results of the large Phase III TOURMALINE MM1 trial, ixazomib has been approved for use in combination with lenalidomide and dexamethasone for the treatment of MM patients who have received at least one prior course of therapy [63].

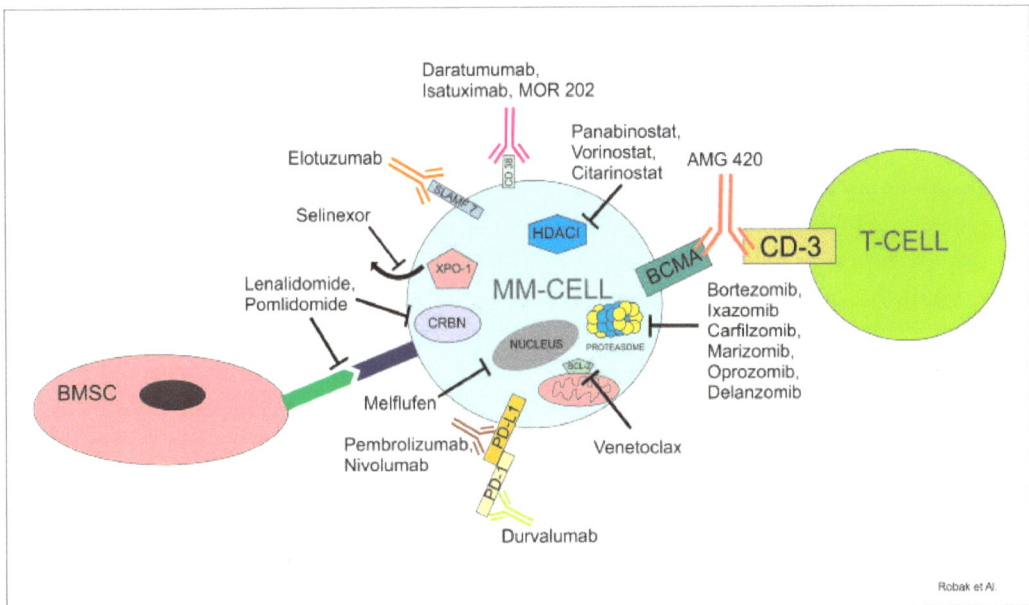

Fig. (1). Schematic presentation of newer drugs for multiple myeloma and their targets. Abbreviatins: BMSC - bone marrow stromal cell; CRBN - cereblon; XPO-1- nuclear export protein exportin- 1 ; SLAMF 7 - SLAM Family Member 7.

4.4. Marizomib

Marizomib (Salinosporamide A, NPI-0052; Triphase ResearchKasaba Hobi, Mysore) is a second-generation beta-lactone-gamma-lactam proteasome inhibitor that inhibits the three proteolytic activities of the 20S proteasome with a specificity distinct from that of bortezomib or carfilzomib [64]. The drug is in clinical development for the treatment of relapsed and refractory MM. The findings of a Phase 1 study indicate that six of 68 tested patients achieved minimal response or better, including five Partial Responses (PR) [65]. The most common Adverse Events (AE) were fatigue, headache, nausea, diarrhea, dizziness and vomiting. The optimal use of marizomib in patients presenting central nervous system AE is described in its patent form [66]. Another study including 14 patients at marizomib, pomalidomide and dexamethasone found six (54%) of 11 evaluable patients to achieve a Partial Response (PR), two (12%) a minimal response and three (27%) Stable Disease (SD) [67].

4.5. Oprazomib

Oprozomib (ONX -0912, Amgen Inc.) is another oral, irreversible PI with a mechanism of action similar to that of marizomib. In a Phase 1b/2 single-agent study performed in 106 patients, PR or better was achieved in 27% of carfilzomib-refractory patients, 33% of carfilzomib-sensitive patients and in 25% of bortezomib-refractory patients [68].

Another Phase 1b/2 study examined the use of oprozomib in combination with dexamethasone in 29 patients with the refractory/relapsed disease [69]. PR was observed in 41.7% of 12 patients receiving oprozomib in doses starting at 210mg per day given on day 1, 2, 8 and 9 of a 14-day cycle; however, no responses were seen when the drug was given on days 1 to 5 of a 14-day cycle. Oprazomib was also tested in combination with pomalidomide and dexamethasone in 31 patients with relapsed/refractory MM [70]. Of 17 patients treated with oprozomib at a dose of 210mg per day on day 1, 2, 8, 9, 15, 16, 22 and 23 of 28-day cycles with subsequent escalations, ten (59%) displayed a PR or better. The combination of oprozomib, pomalidomide and dexamethasone was well tolerated with no major side effects.

4.6. Delanzomib

Delanzomib (CEP-18770, Cephalon, Inc.) is a novel orally-active PI that lowers the activity of NF-κB. It was found to possess a favorable safety profile, with a lack of neurotoxicity [71, 72]. However, a single-agent multicenter Phase 1/2 study of delanzomib in patients with relapsed/refractory MM found that of the patients who received the MTD, 26 (55%) displayed stable disease and four (9%) PR. Median Time to Progression (TTP) was 2.5 months. Due to these disappointing results, further development of delanzomib for MM was discontinued.

4.7. Agents Under Investigation

There are several new proteasome inhibitors currently under investigation, both used alone and in combination with other agents [73 - 75]. Selected recent patents involving novel proteasome inhibitors which may be potentially useful in MM are listed in Table **1** [76 - 80]. Novel spiro- and cyclic bis-benzylidine PIs U pl09 and UP 119 have been developed recently with potential use in MM [73]. Further progress in the treatment of MM has also been made by the combination of proteasome inhibitors with existing therapies [74, 75]. In particular, proteasome-targeting analogs of rapamycin and rapamycin, such as secorapamycin, which are active in bortezomib-resistant cells, have been developed; significantly, secorapamycin acts synergistically *in vitro* with other proteasome inhibitors, including the clinically-approved bortezomib and carfilzomib [76]. Moreover, it has been reported recently that roneparstat, a modified heparin derivative, can increase the antimyeloma activity of bortezomib and carfilzomib [79]. Preclinical and clinical studies have also found that PI activity can be enhanced by co-administration of 17-allylamino-17-demethoxy-geldanamycin or 17-amino geldanamycin [80].

Table 1. Selected Recent Patents Involving Novel Proteasome Inhibitors which may be Potentially Useful in MM.

Inventor	Patent Number	Title	Characteristics	References
Gaczynska, M.E., Osmulski, P.A.	US9918968	Rapamycin analogs targeting proteasome function in the treatment of cancer	Rapamycin and secorapamycin are active in bortezomib resistant MM cells *in vitro* and act synergistically with other PIs, including bortezomib	[76]
Farag, Sherif S.	US20110217258	Combined use of bendamustine, doxorubicin and bortezomib for the treatment of multiple myeloma	Preclinical and clinical studies indicate that bendamustine combined with liposomal doxorubicin and bortezomib is an active regimen for patients with MM	[77]
Chiriva-Internati, M., Figueroa, J.A., Cobos, E.	US20150216931	Galectin-3 inhibitor (GAL-3M) is associated with additive anti-myeloma and anti-solid tumor effects, decreased osteoclastogenesis and organ protection when used in combination with proteasome inhibitors	PIs can be combined with Galectin-3 inhibitor in MM	[74]

(Table 1) contd.....

Inventor	Patent Number	Title	Characteristics	References
Langston, M., Mazaik, D., Elliott, E., Peterson, A., Andres, P., Teng, J.	US20180044356	Novel crystalline form of a proteasome inhibitor	Novel crystalline forms of ixazomib and other boron-containing PIs are reported	[62]
Sanderson, R.D., Ramani, V.P.C., Noseda, A., Barbieri, P.	US20180050061	Roneparstat combined therapy of multiple myeloma	Roneparstat, a modified heparin derivative, can increase the antimyeloma activity of bortezomib and carfilzomib	[79]
Johnson Jr., R.G., Hannah, A.L., Cropp, G.F., Zhou, Y.Q., Sherrill, M.J.	WO2006119032	Method of treating multiple myeloma using 17-AAG or 17-Ag or a prodrug of either in combination with a proteasome inhibitor	PIs displayed synergy when used in combination with 17-allyamino--7-demethoxy-geldanamycin or 17-amino geldanamycin in preclinical and clinical studies	[80]
Chang, Y.-N.	WO2018140907	Novel spiro and cyclic bis-benzylidine proteasome inhibitor for the treatment of cancer, diabetes and neurological disorders	Recently-developed novel spiro and cyclic bis-benzylidine PIs known as UP 109 and UP 119 have potential use in MM	[73]
Trikha, M., Levin, N., Winograd, B.	WO2018169740	Use of a proteasome inhibitor for the treatment of central nervous system cancers	The optimal use of marizomib in patients with adverse events related to the central nervous system	[66]
Reboud-Ravaux, M., Bernard, E., Papapostolou, D., Vanderesse, R.	US20080076718	Novel proteasome modulators		[78]

Abbreviations: MM - Multiple Myeloma; PI - Proteasome Inhibitor

5. IMMUNOMODULATORY DRUGS

Immunomodulatory drugs, also known as IMid compounds, are active in multiple myeloma. Currently, three immunomodulatory drugs, thalidomide, lenalidomide and pomalidomide, are approved for the treatment of MM (Fig. **3**) [81 - 83]. IMiDs target myeloma cells in the BM microenvironment, alter the adhesion of

MM cells to BM stromal cells and directly induce apoptosis or growth arrest of MM cells. Other immunomodulatory effects of IMiDs include inhibition of signaling, through the activity of NFκB, as well as downregulation of the pro-inflammatory cytokine TNF-α and Cyclooxygenase 2 (COX-2). IMiDs have also T-cell co-stimulatory properties, eliminating the requirement for secondary co-stimulation signals from antigen-presenting cells [84 - 86].

They selectively inhibit the production of the pro-inflammatory cytokine TNF-α. IMiDs bind to Cereblon (CRBN), which is a part of the E3 ubiquitin ligase complex and which acts as a substrate receptor of CRL4. These agents trigger a change of CRBN targets, thus initiating therapeutic activity [87].

5.1. Thalidomide

Thalidomide (Thalomid, Celgene) is the first of the IMids, and was used in the late 1950s as a sedative-hypnotic agent [88]. However, congenital malformations associated with ingestion by pregnant women have limited its clinical application for many years [89].

In 1999, thalidomide was found to demonstrate activity against advanced MM which had relapsed after chemotherapy [90]. Thalidomide inhibits the osteoclast-activating factors which promote the osteoclast-activation process and bone pain associated with MM [91]. However, thalidomide is also associated with an unfavorable safety profile, including somnolence, cytopenias and neuropathy.

5.2. Lenalidomide

Lenalidomide (Revlimid, Celgene) is an analog of thalidomide; however it demonstrates more potent antimyeloma activity and lower toxicity than thalidomide [92, 93]. In 2006, the combination of lenalidomide and dexamethasone was first approved by the FDA for the treatment of relapsed/refractory MM. In 2015, this combination was approved for patients with previously untreated MM. Recently, four triplet regimens containing lenalidomide were approved for relapsed/refractory MM: carfilzomib / lenalidomide / dexamethasone; ixazomib / lenalidomide / dexamethasone; elotuzumab / lenalidomide / dexamethasone; daratumumab / lenalidomide / dexamethasone [94]. In previously-untreated MM, better treatment results have been achieved with the use of triple therapy incorporating lenalidomide and a PI. A reduced-dose regimen of lenalidomide/bortezomib/dexamethasone is effective and well tolerated, even in older patients [95]. The two-drug combination of lenalidomide-dexamethasone is also a valid option in previously-treated and relapsed patients.

5.3. Pomalidomide

Pomalidomide (Pomalyst, CC-4047; Imnovid; Celgene Europe Ltd.) is a structural analog of lenalidomide and thalidomide (Fig. **2**). In 2013, EMA approved pomalidomide in combination with dexamethasone for the treatment of patients with relapsed and refractory MM who have received at least two prior treatment regimens, including both lenalidomide and bortezomib, and have demonstrated disease progression during the last course of therapy [96]. Approval was based on the pivotal Phase 3 study (CC-4047-MM-003), whose aim was to compare the efficacy and safety of Pomalidomide combined with Low-Dose Dexamethasone (POM1LoDEX) or with High-Dose Dexamethasone (HiDEX) in relapsed and refractory MM patients who had received at least two prior treatment regimens, including both lenalidomide and bortezomib [97]. Overall response rates were found to be 31% in the bortezomib-refractory patients treated with pomalidomide / dexamethasone but only 13% in the patients receiving high-dose dexamethasone alone; however, median PFS was only 4.0 months and 1.9 months, respectively (p < 0.0001). The OPTIMISMM study, an international Phase 3 trial, was initiated to compare the combination of pomalidomide, bortezomib and dexamethasone (PVD) with that of bortezomib and dexamethasone (VD) in 559 patients with relapsed/refractory MM [56, 98]. The patients had received one or more (median two) lines of prior therapy, but had to show response to proteasome inhibitors. PVD was found to be superior to VD: after a median follow-up of 16 months, PVD significantly reduced the risk of progression or death by 39% in comparison with VD. PVD and VD treatment yielded respective Overall Response (OR) rates of 82.2% and 50.0%, and PFS values of 11.2 months and 7.10 months. Similarly, the respective OR rates were 85.9% and 50.8% in lenalidomide-refractory patients, and 95.7% and 60.0% in lenalidomide-nonrefractory patients. Median PFS values were 17.8 months for PVD and 9.5 months for VD in lenalidomide-refractory patients, and 22.0 months compared to 12.0 months in lenalidomide-nonrefractory patients.

5.4. Agents Under Investigation

There is currently great interest in identifying new approaches to IMid use, and some of these are the subject of recent patents (Table **2**). For example, the combination of Histone Deacetylases (HDAC)Histone Deacetylases (HDACs) deacetylate the lysine residues of histones and inhibitors or proteasome inhibitors and IMids can act synergistically in promoting neoplastic cell killing [99, 100].

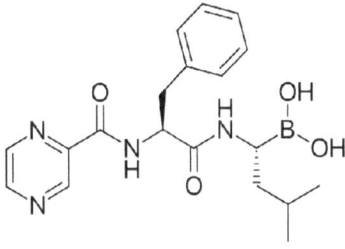

Bortezomib

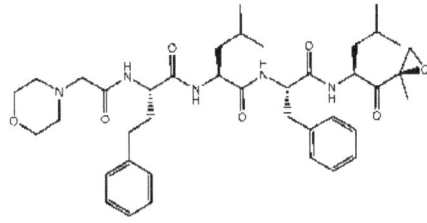

Carfilzomib

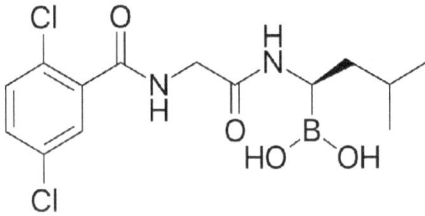

Ixazomib

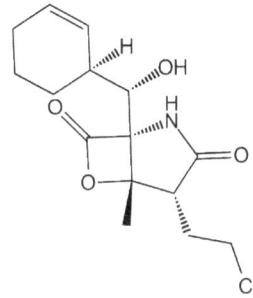

Marizomib

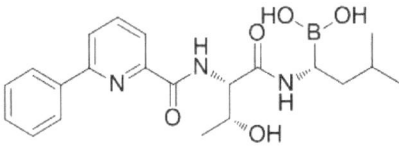

Delanzomib

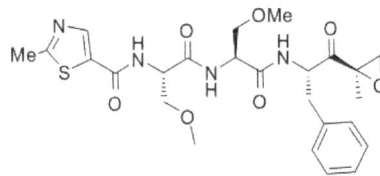

Oprozomib

Fig. (2). Chemical structures of proteasome inhibitors.

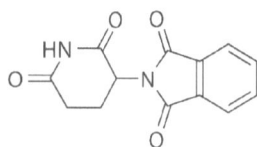

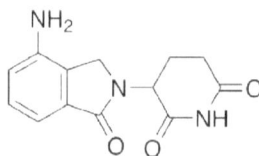

| Thalidomide | Lenalidomide | Pomalidomide |

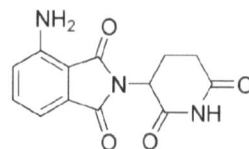

Fig. (3). Chemical structures of immunomodulatory drugs.

Table 2. Recent Patents Involving Novel Immunomodulatory Drugs with Potential Value in Treating MM.

Inventor	Patent Number	Title	Characteristics	References
Quayle, S.N., Jones, S.S.	US9949972	Combinations of histone deacetylase inhibitors and immunomodulatory drugs	The combination of HDAC inhibitors and IMids can act synergistically in the promotion of neoplastic cell apoptosis	[100]
Lara Ochoa, J.M.	WO2010008263	Use of thalidomide to inhibit the osteoclast-activation process associated with multiple myeloma disease	Thalidomide inhibits the osteoclast-activating factors which promote osteoclast activation, decrease bone pain and decrease fractures associated with MM	[91]

Abbreviations: HDAC - Histone Deacetylase; IMids - Immunomodulatory drugs ; MM - Multiple Myeloma

6. HISTONE DEACETYLASE INHIBITORS

Histone Deacetylases deacetylate the lysine residues of histones and other proteins [101, 102]. HDAC inhibitors can be divided into two classes, those that inhibit both Class I (HDAC1-3 and 8) and IIb (HDAC6 and 10) enzymes and those that inhibit Class I enzymes alone [103]. Preclinical and clinical studies have found the combination of HDAC inhibitors with PIs or IMiDs to show significant activity. The Pan-HDAC inhibitors vorinostat and panobinostat have been approved by the FDA for the treatment of relapsed/refractory MM (Fig. **4**); however, their clinical value is limited due to poor tolerability.

6.1. Vorinostat

Vorinostat (Zolinza, Merck) is an oral class I/II HDAC inhibitor. This agent has been investigated in combination with bortezomib in the VANTAGE088 randomized Phase 3 trial performed in relapsed and refractory MM patients [104].

Median PFS was found to be 7.6 months for vorinostat and bortezomib and 6.8 months for bortezomib-control. Vorinostat, Bortezomib, Doxorubicin and Dexamethasone (VBDD/VERUMM) were also evaluated in 33 relapsed and refractory patients with MM [105]. With a median follow-up of 30.8 months, median PFS was 9.6 months and OS 33.8 months. In a Phase 2b study, vorinostat was combined with lenalidomide and dexamethasone in 25 lenalidomide-refractory MM patients [106]. Vorinostat was given orally at 400mg/day on days 1-7 and 15-21, lenalidomide at 25 mg on days 1-21, and dexamethasone at 40mg on days 1, 8, 15 and 22 in 28-day cycles. The OR rate was 24%, the median duration of response was three months and the median PFS was 5.3 months.

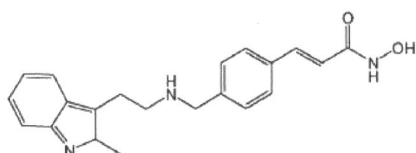

Panobinostat   Vorinostat

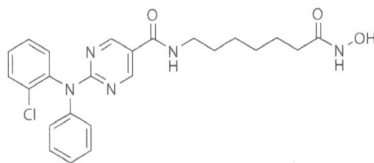

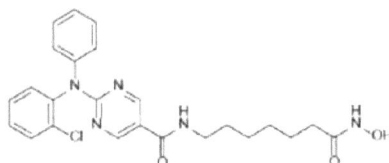

Citarinostat   Ricolinostat

Fig. (4). Chemical structure of histone deacetylase inhibitors.

6.2. Panobinostat

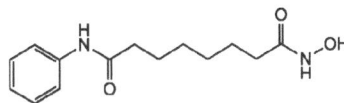

Panobinostat (Farydak, Novartis) is an orally-available HDAC inhibitor. It is the first HDAC inhibitor approved for MM. The limited activity was observed with panobinostat monotherapy in MM patients. In a Phase 2 trial of 38 patients, only one partial response lasting 19 months and one minimal response lasting 28 months were observed [107, 108]. Panobinostat was approved by EMA in combination with bortezomib and dexamethasone for the treatment of MM patients with relapsed and/or refractory disease who have received at least two prior regimens including bortezomib and immunomodulatory agents [109]. Approval was based on the results of the PANORAMA-1 trial comparing a panobinostat/bortezomib/ dexamethasone regimen with one based on bortezomib/dexamethasone/ placebo in patients with relapsed/refractory MM [110, 111]. This Phase 3 trial was performed in 768 patients with relapsed or relapsed and refractory MM who had received one to three prior lines of therapies. In the subgroup of patients who had received at least two prior regimens including bortezomib and an IMid, PFS was 12.5 months for the experimental arm and 4.7 months for the control arm (p = 0 .0003). The high-risk patients in the panobinostat arm tended to display a longer OS (33.3 months) than those in the placebo arm (22.8 months); however, the high risk and standard-risk patients in the panobinostat arm displayed similar OS values (35.0 months) [112]. The occurrence of grade 3-4 AE associated with the study drug was 76.9% for the panobinostat group and 51.2% for the placebo group. The most common grade 3-4 severe AEs associated with panobinostat were diarrhea (18.9%), fatigue (14.7%), nausea (4.5%), vomiting (5.5%), thrombocytopenia (43.6%), anemia (7.9%), neutropenia (16.5%) and lymphopenia (8.1%). The patients with relapsed MM enrolled on the Myeloma UK (MUK)-six Phase I/II trial demonstrated a median overall PFS of 16.1 months following a course of low-dose thalidomide, low-intensity subcutaneous bortezomib and dexamethasone followed by panobinostat maintenance [113].

6.3. Ricolinostat

Ricolinostat (ACY-1215, Celgene) is the first selective orally-available selective HDAC6 inhibitor with reduced class I HDAC activity showing anti-myeloma efficacy in combination with proteasome inhibitors [114, 115]. In a Phase 1/2 trial, ricolinostat was used in combination with bortezomib and dexamethasone in patients with relapsed or refractory MM. Therapy was well tolerated, with less severe hematologic and gastrointestinal toxicities compared with nonselective HDAC inhibitors. The OR rate was 37% in all the patients and 14% in bortezomib-refractory patients when ricolinostat was administered at ≥ 160mg daily [114]. Ricolinostat was also investigated in combination with lenalidomide and dexamethasone in relapsed or refractory MM in a multicentre Phase 1b trial [116]. The response was observed in 21 (55%) of 38 patients. The most common AEs were fatigue and diarrhea.

6.4. Citarinostat

Citarinostat (ACY-241, Acetylon Pharmaceuticals) is the second generation selective HDAC6 inhibitor with a more favorable safety profile than non-selective pan-HDAC inhibitors. Preclinical studies demonstrate the synergy between citarinostat and pomalidomide in both *in vitro* and *in vivo* models, providing further rationale for clinical development of the combined use of these agents [117].

6.5. Agents Under Investigation

Several new HDAC inhibitors are under investigation in neoplastic diseases, either alone or in combination with other agents (Table **3**). PXD-101 (Belinostat) was investigated in combination with dexamethasone, bortezomib, thalidomide, vincristine, doxorubicin and melphalan on the U26 myeloma cell line [118, 119]. A method for testing whether a patient with MM will respond to HDACi has recently been reported in the patent form [120]. In addition, several new molecules with HDACi activity are reported [121].

Table 3. Recent Patents Involving Novel Histone Deacetylase Inhibitors with Potential Value in Treating MM.

Inventor	Patent Number	Title	Drug Characteristics	References
Lichenstein, H., Jeffers, M., Qian, X., Sehested, M., Peterson, K.D., Ritchie, J.	US20150231096	Combination therapies using HDAC inhibitors	PXD-101 (Belinostat) was investigated in combination with dexamethasone in a U266 myeloma cell line	[118]
Lichenstein, H., Edwards, N., Ritchie, J., Erichsen, K.D., Plumb, J.	US20180271852	(Histone Deacetylase (HDAC) inhibitors for the treatment of cancer.) inhibitors for the treatment of cancer	PXD-101 (Belinostat) was investigated in combination with bortezomib, thalidomide, vincristine, doxorubicin and melphalan	[119]
Moreaux, J., Klein, B.	US20150275305	Methods for predicting multiple myeloma treatment response	Method for testing whether a patient with MM will respond to HDACi	[120]
Stuttleworth, S.J., Tomassi, C.D., Cecil, A.R.L., MacCormick, S., Nodes, W.J., Silva, F.A.	US20180170876	Novel histone deacetylase inhibitors	Several new molecules with HDACi activity are reported	[121]

Abbreviations: HDACi - Histone Deacetylase inhibitor; MM - Multiple Myeloma

7. MONOCLONAL ANTIBODIES

An important new strategy is based on the use of monoclonal antibodies against target antigens expressed on MM cells. Two of these antibodies, elotuzumab and daratumumab, have recently been approved for the treatment of MM. Mabs acting as anti-PD1 checkpoint inhibitors have also been investigated in MM.

7.1. Daratumumab

Daratumumab (Darzalex, Janssen) is a humanized IgG1 anti-CD38 antibody with direct on-tumor and immunomodulatory mechanisms of action [122]. The anti-myeloma activity of daratumumab is mediated by Antibody-Dependent Cellular Cytotoxicity (ADCC), Complement-Dependent Cytotoxicity (CDC), macrophage-mediated phagocytosis and apoptosis via Fc-mediated crosslinking [123, 124]. Daratumumab induces the recruitment of effector cells and removal of CD38+ immune-suppressor cells, and exerts direct apoptotic activity. In addition, daratumumab induces rapid internalization of CD38 on the surface of MM cells and impairs MM cell adhesion. It also potentiates the killing of MM cells by bortezomib *in vitro* and *in vivo*, independent of its function as an immune activator [125].

Daratumumab is active in previously-untreated and heavily-pretreated relapsed or refractory MM patients [126 - 130]. The addition of daratumumab to lenalidomide and dexamethasone significantly prolonged PFS among patients with relapsed or refractory MM [129]. In the POLLUX trial, the PFS at 12 months was found to be 83.2% in patients treated with daratumumab, lenalidomide and dexamethasone and 60.1% in patients treated with lenalidomide and dexamethasone only; approximately 86% of the studied patients had been previously treated with bortezomib, and 20% were refractory to PIs [129]. Another large randomized study performed in patients with relapsed and/or refractory MM yielded a higher OR among patients treated with bortezomib/dexamethasone/ daratumumab (89.2%) than those receiving bortezomib/dexamethasone (63.2%); in addition, PFS at 12 months was 60.7% in the daratumumab arm and 26.9% in the control group [128]. Daratumumab in combination with pomalidomide and dexamethasone has also been investigated in a Phase 2 study in patients refractory to both lenalidomide and bortezomib: the OR rate was approximately 90% in patients who were naïve to daratumumab and pomalidomide [130]. This combination has been approved by the FDA. Recently, the combination of daratumumab with bortezomib, melphalan and prednisone was approved in the United States for patients with newly-diagnosed MM who are unsuitable for ASCT. This approval was based on the results of a large randomized study (Alcyone) comparing daratumumab + VTP (bortezomib, melphalan, and prednisone) with VTP alone in 706 patients with the newly diagnosed MM who were ineligible for ASCT [131]. The OR rate was 90.9% in the daratumumab group and 73.9% in the control group, with CR rates of 42.6% and 24.4%, respectively (P < 0.001). The 18-month PFS rate was 71.6% in the VTP + daratumumab group and 50.2% in the VTP group at a median follow-up of 16.5 months, (P < 0.001). Infusion reactions and infections are the most common Adverse Events (AE) in MM patients treated with daratumumab [132]. Among 348 patients treated with this agent in an early access treatment protocol, serious AEs were noted in 35% of patients and 12% were drug-related. During the first infusions, reactions occurred in 56% of cases and infections in 11%.

7.2. Isatuximab

Isatuximab (SAR650984; Sanofi) is a humanized IgG1 mAb directed to a specific epitope on the human CD38 receptor with clinical activity in heavily pretreated patients with MM [133]. Isatuximab was evaluated in monotherapy in 84 patients with relapsed/refractory MM as part of Phase 1 dose-escalation study [134]. The Maximum Tolerated Dose (MTD) was not reached and no cumulative adverse reactions were noted. The most frequently-observed infusion reactions were Treatment-Emergent Adverse Events (TEAEs), and these were observed in 51% of patients, despite mandatory prophylaxis. The most frequent grade 3/4 hematologic abnormalities were lymphopenia (34%), anemia (20%), thrombocytopenia (17%) and neutropenia (12%). Other common TEAEs included fatigue (37%), nausea (32%), upper respiratory tract infection (24%), and coughing (23%). Among the patients receiving isatuximab ≥ 10mg/kg, OR Rate (ORR) was found to be 23.8%, and CR was observed in one patient. The median duration of response at doses ≥ 10mg/kg was 25 weeks among high-risk patients, compared to 36 weeks for other patients. The combination of isatuximab, lenalidomide and dexamethasone is also active and well tolerated in heavily-pretreated patients with MM: a Phase 1b, open-label, dose-escalation study found the OR rate to be 56% and median PFS 8.5 months [135]. Recently, a Phase 1b dose-escalation study evaluated isatuximab combined with pomalidomide and dexamethasone in 45 patients with relapsed/refractory MM. As reported by Mikhael *et al.*, the OR rate was 62% with a median duration of response 18.7 months and median PFS was 17.6 months. The most common adverse events were fatigue (62%), upper respiratory tract infection (42%), infusion reactions (42%), and dyspnea (40%) [136].

7.3. Elotuzumab

Elotuzumab (BMS986015, Empliciti, Bristol-Myers Squibb), is a humanized mAb directed against Signaling Lymphocytic Activation Molecule F7 (SLAMF7). The drug induces ADCC and exerts stimulatory effects on NK cells, which are mediated by the engagement of elotuzumab with SLAMF7 [137]. It has been approved for the treatment of relapsed or refractory MM. The combination of elotuzumab, lenalidomide and dexamethasone has been found to offer 30% higher PFS and OS than lenalidomide/dexamethasone alone in a group of previously-treated MM patients, 70% of whom were previously exposed to bortezomib [138]. Elotuzumab is also an active drug in patients with MM who had previously been treated with bortezomib.

7.4. MOR202

MOR202 is a human mAb directed against CD38 in clinical development for the treatment of MM. MOR202 is currently under clinical investigation in a Phase 1/2a, open-label, multicenter, dose-escalation study, both alone and in combination with pomalidomide/lenalidomide/ dexamethasone, in patients with relapsed/refractory MM (NCT01421186).

7.5. Pembrolizumab

Pembrolizumab (Keytruda, MK-3475, Merck) is a highly-selective humanized anti-PD1 checkpoint-inhibitor mAb. A Phase 1b clinical trial evaluated Pembrolizumab as a single drug, administered at a dose of 10mg/kg every two weeks or at a set dose of 200mg every three weeks, in 30 relapsed/refractory MM patients with a median of 4 previous lines of therapy [139]. Seventeen (57%) patients demonstrated stable disease but no patients achieved a response. In addition, 13 (43%) patients had progressive disease. Treatment-related AEs occurred in 12 (40%) patients, including asthenia, arthralgia, increased aspartate aminotransferase, fatigue, hyperglycemia, hypothyroidism, myalgia, pruritus and blurred vision; however, only one grade 3 AE was observed related to treatment, and this was myalgia.

Pembrolizumab is also undergoing evaluation in combination with lenalidomide / dexamethasone or pomalidomide / dexamethasone [140]. In this Phase 2 study including 48 patients with relapsed/refractory MM, pembrolizumab was given at a dose of 200mg IV every two weeks, pomalidomide at 4mg daily for 21 days, and dexamethasone 40mg weekly. Overall responses were observed in 29 of 48 (60%) patients, including four CR (8%), nine Very Good PR (VGPR) (19%), and 16 (33%) PR. Median response duration was 14.7 months and median PFS was 17.4 months. Most common grade 3 and 4 AEs were hematologic toxicities (40%), hyperglycemia (25%) and pneumonia (15%). The KEYNOTE-185 study compared the safety and efficacy of pembrolizumab with that of lenalidomide and dexamethasone in 301 previously-untreated MM patients: the relative risk of death in the pembrolizumab arm (19 deaths) was more than twice to that observed in the control group (nine deaths) at the median follow-up of 6.6 months [141].

7.6. Nivolumab

Nivolumab (Opdivo, MDX1106, BMS-936558, Bristol-Myers Squibb) is a fully human IgG4 anti-PD1 mAb. Leshokin *et al.* have published the results of a Phase 1 clinical trial assessing nivolumab as a single agent in 27 patients with relapsed or refractory T- or B-cell lymphoma or MM treated with nivolumab [142]. Stable disease was observed in 17/27 (63%) and no better responses were observed.

7.7. Durvalumab

Durvalumab is a human IgG1k antibody targeting PD-L1 and blocking its interaction with PD-1 and CD80 [143]. A Phase 1/2 study of durvalumab in combination with lenalidomide, with and without dexamethasone, in patients with newly-diagnosed multiple myeloma is ongoing (ClinicalTrials.gov Identifier: NCT02685826).

7.8. Agents Under Investigation

Several new mAbs with anti-myeloma activity are under investigation in preclinical and clinical studies (Table **4**). HuLuc63 has demonstrated antimyeloma activity in SCID mice with OPM2 MM cells, as well as synergy with bortezomib in the preclinical study, and currently under investigation in a Phase 1b study in combination with bortezomib or lenalidomide / dexamethasone [144]. New human anti-CD38 mAbs inducing CDC-mediated lysis of CD38-transfected CHO cells have been disclosed recently in the patent form [145]. In addition, recent patents also discuss the use of mAbs and small molecules to modulate the immune response modulation by targeting ABCB5 and immune checkpoint molecule-related pathways [146].

8. OTHER AGENTS

Several other agents with various chemical structures and mechanisms of action have been presented in recent years.

8.1. Dinaciclib

Dinaciclib (MK-7965, SCH 727965; Merck/Ligand Pharmaceuticals) is a potent and specific inhibitor of Cyclin-Dependent Kinases (CDK) CDK1, CDK2, CDK5, and CDK9 which interacts with the acetyl-lysine recognition site of bromodomains and inhibits the unfolded protein response through a CDK1 and CDK5-dependent mechanism [147]. Preclinical studies found dinaciclib/doxorubicin to inhibit the growth of MM RPMI-8226 cells and promote senescence by transforming the suppressive effects of the ATM/Chk2/p53/p21 signaling pathway and enhancing the p16 signaling pathway [148]. An initial Phase 1/2 single-agent open-label trial conducted on 27 relapsed patients yielded an OR rate of 18.5% including three (11%) PR or better and two minimal responses [149]. The most common hematologic AEs were diarrhea (87%), fatigue (67%), thrombocytopenia (60%), nausea (53%) and leukopenia (27%).

Table 4. Recent Patents Involving Novel Monoclonal Antibodies with Potential Value in Treating MM.

Inventor	Patent Number	Title	Drug characteristics	References
Afar, D., Andersen, K.C., Tai, Y.-T.	EP3115049	Combination therapies based on anti-CS1 antibodies for treating multiple myeloma	In the preclinical study, the HuLuc63 mAb showed antimyeloma activity in SCID mice with OPM2 MM cells, and synergy with bortezomib. In the Phase 1b study, HuLuc63 mAb is investigated in combination with bortezomib or with lenalidomide and dexamethasone	[144]
De Weers, M., Graus, Y., Oprins, J., Parren, P., Van De, W.J., Van Vugt, M.	EP3312196	Antibodies against CD38 for treatment of multiple myeloma	New human anti-CD38 mAbs with anti-MM activity are described	[145]
Nandabalan, K., Sharma, H., Sapra, A.K., Upmanyu, S.	US20180134771	Novel immunomodulatory therapeutic strategies targeting tumors in cancer	Modulation of the immune response by targeting ABCB5 and pathways related to an immune checkpoint molecule using mAbs and small molecules	[146]

Abbreviations: mAbs- monoclonal Antibodies; MM - Multiple Myeloma

8.2. Filanesib

Filanesib (ARRY-520, Array BioPharma (Boulder, CO, USA) is a highly selective inhibitor of Kinesin Spindle Protein (KSP). KSP plays a role in the separation of spindle poles and the generation of bipolar spindles in mitosis [150]. It was investigated as a single agent as part of a Phase 1 / 2 study in patients with relapsed/refractory MM, and later, in combination with dexamethasone in Phase 2 expansion cohorts [151]. The most common dose-limiting toxicities are grade 3 and 4 cytopenias, observed in approximately 50% of patients. Partial responses were noted in 16% of patients when filanesib was used as a single agent and 15% when combined with dexamethasone [152].

8.3. Trametinib

Trametinib (GSK1120212, Mekinist) is a reversible inhibitor of MEK1/MEK2 activation and MEK1/MEK2 kinase activity. Trametinib is approved by the US FDA as a single agent or in combination with dabrafenib for the treatment of unresectable or metastatic melanoma with a BRAF V600E/V600K mutation. In a Phase 1 study, one PR was reported and four patients demonstrated SD as the best response [153]. The most common adverse events were diarrhea (60%), dermatitis (55%), maculopapular rash (45%), fatigue (30%), dry skin (25%), nausea (25%), dyspnea (20%), and vomiting (20%).

8.4. Afuresertib

Afuresertib (PKB115125; GSK2110183, Novartis) is a novel ATP-competitive inhibitor mainly targeting the ATP binding and subsequent phosphorylation of Akt substrates. This agent has clinical activity in monotherapy against several hematological malignancies. Afuresertib is expected to be used in combination with standard therapies for MM. In preclinical studies, it demonstrated single-agent clinical activity. In addition, it exerts synergistic anti-myeloma effects against MM cell lines, with low sensitivity to both pomalidomide and afuresertib monotherapies [154]. Single-agent afuresertib showed a favorable safety profile and demonstrated some clinical efficacy in MM patients [155]. In an open-label Phase 1 study, 73 patients were treated at doses ranging from 25 to 150mg per day. The MTD was established at 125mg per day. Three MM myeloma obtained a PR, while three attained minimal responses. The most frequent AEs were nausea (35.6%), diarrhea (32.9%) and dyspepsia (24.7%).

8.5. LGH447

LGH447 (Novartis Pharmaceuticals) is a pan-PIM (Provirus Integration site for

Moloney leukemia) kinase inhibitor which has been tested preclinically and in clinical trials in MM [156]. Preclinical studies indicate a dose-dependent decrease in cell proliferation in a majority of tested MM cell lines. In a Phase 1 study, LGH447 was well tolerated and exhibited evidence of single-agent efficacy, with a response being observed in 20.8% of 54 heavily-pretreated patients with MM, including one VGPR and four PRs. Five additional patients achieved Minimal Response (MR) and 23 patients had SD. The most common AEs were thrombocytopenia (19%), anemia (19%), neutropenia (13%) and fatigue (11%) [157].

8.6. Venetoclax

Venetoclax (Venclexta, AbbVie) is an oral BCL-2 inhibitor which shows high activity in the treatment of B-cell malignancies. Preclinical studies have found venetoclax to enhance bortezomib activity, suggesting that such a combination could be an effective one in the treatment of MM. Although it has been demonstrated to show some activity as monotherapy of MM patients with t(11;14) [158 - 162], venetocax is more active when given in combination with bortezomib/dexamethasone: this combination was found to achieve PR in 67% of patients, including 78% of those with t(11;14) and who express high levels of BCL-2 relative to BCL-X_L and MCL-1 [159]. Elsewhere, the four-drug combination of venetoclax, bortezomib, daratumumab and dexamethasone was found to yield a CR in two heavily-pretreated patients [160]. In a Phase 1b trial performed in 66 patients with relapsed/refractory MM, venetoclax was used at a dose of 50-1200mg per day in combination with bortezomib and dexamethasone [159]. The treatment was tolerated, and most common adverse events were mild gastrointestinal toxicities, constipation, nausea and grade 3/4 cytopenias. The OR Rate was 67% including 42% good partial response or better with median time to progression 9.5 months and duration of response 9.7 months.

A Phase 1 study of 66 patients with relapsed/refractory MM treated with venetoclax monotherapy [163]; 61% of the patients were double refractory to bortezomib and lenalidomide and 46% had t(11;14). The OR rate was 21% (14/66), and 15% achieved VGPR or better. In the patients with t(11;14), the OR rate was 86%. Most common AEs were nausea (47%), diarrhea (36%), vomiting (21%), thrombocytopenia (32%), neutropenia (27%), and anemia (23%). In an ongoing Phase 2, dose escalation study, patients with refractory/relapsed MM were treated with Venetoclax combined with carfilzomib and dexamethasone [164]. The OR rate was found to be 78%, including a 56% VGPR or better. Patients with t(11;14) demonstrated the most favourable response: OR rate 100% and VGPR 88%.

8.7. Melflufen

Melflufen (Melphalan flufenamide ethyl ester, Ygalo, Oncopeptides, AB) is a peptidase-potentiated alkylating drug which rapidly penetrates target cells. In aminopeptidase-positive cells, the drug undergoes enzymatic cleavage, allowing high intracellular concentrations of its metabolite ranging from 10- to 100-fold to be achieved. This agent is a more potent anti-MM agent than melphalan. Melflufen induces irreversible DNA damage and may overcome melphalan-resistance in MM cells [165, 166]. In addition, melflufen has potent anti-angiogenic properties and overcomes conventional drug resistance [139]. Melflufen may also possess greater efficacy and less toxicity than melphalan [166]. In a Phase 2 study, 40mg melflufen was given i.v. on day 1 of each 28-day cycle, with 40mg dexamethasone weekly, in 45 relapsed or refractory MM patients with two or more prior lines of therapy including lenalidomide and bortezomib [167]. The OR rate was 41%, including four patients with VGPR (12%) and ten with PR (29%). Seven (21%) additional patients achieved a minimal response, for a clinical benefit rate of 62%. The median PFS for all treated patients was 5.1 months. In patients with PR or higher, the PFS was 11.0 months. The median OS in all treated patients was 20.7 months. The most frequent all-grades AEs were thrombocytopenia (76%), anemia (62%) and neutropenia (60%). Melflufen was also investigated in a Phase 1/2 study in MM patients refractory to daratumumab and/or pomalidomide [168]. The OR rate was found to be 32% among a total of 56 patients evaluable for response. Treatment-related grade 3/4 AEs were neutropenia (60%), thrombocytopenia (60%), and anemia (27%). Grade 3/4 infections were observed in 6% of patients.

8.8. Selinexor

Selinexor (Karyopharm Therapeutics) is an oral inhibitor of the nuclear export protein exportin 1 (XPO1), which has yielded promising results in refractory MM, including patients resistant to daratumumab [169]. This agent induces apoptosis of neoplastic cells through nuclear retention of tumor suppressor proteins and inhibits the translation of oncoprotein mRNAs, and is thought to force reactivation of cell cycle regulators such as p53, IkB, and Rb. Preclinical studies have found the combination of selinexor and PIs to display synergistic antimyeloma activity by suppression of NFκB signaling and nuclear retention of tumor suppressor proteins. Similarly, the combination of selinexor with IMiDs has also shown synergistic anti-MM activity in murine MM models.

A Phase 1 study was performed in 22 heavily-pretreated patients with MM and three patients with Waldenstrom macroglobulinemia [170]. In the dose-expansion phase, 59 patients with MM received selinexor at 45 or $60mg/m^2$ with 20mg dexamethasone, twice weekly in 28-day cycles, or selinexor (40 or 60mg flat dose) without corticosteroids in 21-day cycles. The most common nonhematologic AEs were nausea (75%), fatigue (70%), anorexia (64%), vomiting (43%), weight loss (32%), and diarrhea (32%), which were primarily grade 1 or 2. The most common grade 3 or 4 AEs were hematologic, particularly thrombocytopenia (45%). Single-agent selinexor demonstrated modest efficacy, with an OR rate of 4% and a clinical benefit rate of 21%. Higher OR rates were observed for selinexor and dexamethasone; all responses of PR or better were observed in the 45mg/m^2 selinexor plus 20mg dexamethasone twice weekly cohort (OR rate - 50%). Furthermore, 46% of all patients showed a reduction in MM markers from baseline. These findings indicate that selinexor in combination with dexamethasone is active in heavily-pretreated MM.

A Phase 2 trial examined the effect of combined selinexor and dexamethasone administration in 78 patients with highly-refractory MM with a median of seven prior regimens based on the most active available agents [171]. Most of the patients had high-risk cytogenetics, including t(4;14), t(14;16), and del(17p). OR rate was 35% (six of 17 patients). The OR rate was 21%, and 65% of responded patients survived to at least 12 months, with a median duration of response of five months. The most common grade $\geq$ 3 AEs were thrombocytopenia (59%), anemia (28%), neutropenia (23%), hyponatremia (22%), leukopenia (15%), and fatigue (15%).

In the STORM study, 122 patients with penta-refractory MM were treated with 8mg selinexor plus 20mg dexamethasone twice weekly [172]. The OR rate ($\geq$ PR) was 26.2%, with 6.5% $\geq$ VGPR, including 2 CR. Responses typically occurred within the first month and median PFS was 3.7 months, and OS 8.0 months. The most frequently-reported treatment-related all-grades AEs were thrombocytopenia (67%), nausea (67%), fatigue (68%), anorexia (50%), anemia (46%) and weight loss (46%).

Selinexor was also tested in combination with low-dose bortezomib and dexamethasone in 42 relapsed or refractory MM. The OR rates were 63% for all the patients, 84% for PI-non-refractory patients and 43% for PI-refractory patients, while the median PFS values were 9.0 months for all the patients, 17.8 months for PI-non-refractory and 6.1 months for PI-refractory [173]. Elsewhere, a study of 34 patients with relapsed or refractory MM who had received $\geq$ two prior therapies including lenalidomide and a PI [174] found the combination of selinexor and pomalidomide to yield OR rates of 55% among lenalidomide-relapsed or refractory patients and 38% among pomalidomide and lenalidomide-refractory patients. Median PFS was 10.3 months with a median follow up of 9.4 months.

8.9. Sphingosine Kinase 2 Inhibitors

Sphingosine Kinase 2 (SK2) is an enzyme that catalyses the formation of the bioactive lipid, Sphingosine 1-Phosphate (S1P). SK2 is overexpressed in MM cell lines and in human MM cells and plays a critical role in myeloma cell growth, proliferation and survival. This kinase can be a target for anti-MM drugs [175]. ABC294640 (Opaganib, YELIVA®, RedHill Biopharma Ltd.) is a novel SK2 selective inhibitor with a possibly unique mechanism of action that has shown promising preclinical activity. ABC294640 induces apoptosis in primary human CD138+ cells and MM cell lines [176]. It also promotes proteasome degradation of Mcl-1 and c-Myc and inhibits myeloma growth *in vitro* and *in vivo*. In addition, ABC294640 and venetoclax exhibit synergistic antimyeloma activity *in vitro* and *in vivo* in myeloma cells without a t(11;14) translocation [177]. The findings of a Phase Ib study with single agent ABC294640 in relapsed/refractory myeloma were presented at the EORTC conference: no dose-limiting toxicities were reported, and two of 10 evaluable patients had stable disease for over four months, with one patient achieving VGPR [178].

8.10. Bispecific T Cell Engager (BiTE®) Antibodies

Bispecific T cell Engager (BiTE®) antibodies bind concomitantly to T cells and tumor cells, whereupon they induce selective cytolytic activity in T cells against neoplastic cells [179]. Hipp *et al*. developed a novel BCMA BiTE® antibody known as AMG420 (BI 836909; Amgen) targeting B Cell Maturation Antigen (BCMA) and CD3ε and investigated its influence on MM cells [180]. BI 836909 caused selective lysis of BCMA-positive MM cells and activation of T cells; it also induced cytokine release and T cell proliferation. In *ex vivo* experiments, BI 836909 induced the lysis of autologous MM cells in samples collected from previously-untreated and relapsed/refractory MM patients. In mouse xenograft studies based on an orthotopic L-363 xenograft model with subcutaneous NCI-H929 xenografts, BI 836909 induced tumor cell depletion and prolonged survival.

The maximum tolerated dose and dose-limiting toxicities of AMG 420 in relapsed or refractory multiple myeloma patients, and in those who demonstrated progression after ≥ 2 prior treatment lines, were examined as part of a Phase 1 trial (NCT02514239) conducted in France and Germany [181]. Thirty-five patients received AMG 420 at doses ranging from 0.2 to 800μg/d. Six patients achieved CR and two reached PR. Importantly, all three patients with CRs at 400μg/d were MRD negative. No major toxicities were observed up to 400μg/d, which is the recommended dose for further studies. These results indicate that AMG 420 shows potential as a new antimyeloma drug, and supports its further investigation in clinical studies in MM patients.

8.11. Novel Agents Reported in the Patent Forms

Glutaminase is a potential therapeutic target in MM cells. Heterocyclic inhibitors of glutaminase with antimyeloma activity have been developed recently (Table **5**) [182]; however, their clinical value is presently unknown. Carboline derivatives that inhibit NF-kB are also believed to demonstrate potential therapeutic activity in MM, and have been found to inhibit the growth of MM cell lines [183]. For example, compound 1 inhibits NF-kB activation and decreases the viability of MM cell lines; it also has been found to induce G1 growth arrest in U266 and RPM18226 cell lines.

Other agents known to possess antimyeloma properties include the topotecan derivative HM910, that has been found to inhibit the growth of NCI-H929 MM xenografts in nude mice [184], and 4-(4-fluoro-2-methoxyphenyl)-N-{3-[(s-methylsulfonimidoyl)methyl] phenyl}-1,3,5-triazin-2-amine, which has displayed high activity in an NCI-H929 MM xenograft model subcutaneously implanted into NOD/SCI mice [185]. Novel bicyclic bromodomain inhibitors have also demonstrated *in vivo* antimyeloma activity in an MM xenograft model based on MM1.s cells in an athymic nude mouse strain [186]. Finally, antagonists of 4 integrin/alpha 4 integrin ligand adhesion have shown promise in suppressing the bone destruction associated with MM [187].

Table 5. Selected Patents Involving Other Drugs with Potential Value in Treating MM.

Inventor	Patent Number	Title	Drug Characteristics	References
MacKinnon, A.L., Rodriguez, M.L.	WO2016014890	Treatment of multiple myeloma with heterocyclic inhibitors of glutaminase	Heterocyclic inhibitors of glutaminase with antimyeloma activity are presented	[182]
Adams, J.	WO2003039545	Carboline derivatives as inhibitors of IKB in the treatment of multiple myeloma and others cancers	Some carboline derivatives inhibit the growth of MM cell lines and have potential in MM treat-ment. Compound 1 inhibits NF-kB activation and decreases the viability of MM cell lines. It also induces G1 growth arrest in U266 and RPM18226 cell lines	[183]
Deng, J.	EP3100734	Use of camptothecin derivative in preparing pharmaceutical used for treating multiple myeloma	Topotecan derivative HM910 displays significant anti-myeloma efficacy against MM cell NCI-H9 29 xenografts in nude mice	[184]
Scholz, A.	US20180078560	Use of 4-(4-fluoro-2-methoxyphenyl)- N-{3-[(S-methyl sulfonimidoyl)methyl]phenyl}-1,3,5-triazin-2-amine for treating multiple myeloma	High anti-myeloma activity was observed for 4-(4-fluoro-2-methoxyphenyl)-N-{3-[(S-meth ylsulfonimidoyl)methyl]phenyl}-1,3,5-triazin-2-amine in an NCI-H929 MM xenograft model subcutaneously implanted into NOD/SCI mice	[185]

(Table 5) contd.....

Inventor	Patent Number	Title	Drug Characteristics	References
Quinn, J.F., Duffy, B.C., Liu, S., Wang, R., Jiang, M.X., Martin, G.S., Wagner, G.S., Young, P.R.	US20180161337	Novel bicyclic bromodomain inhibitors	Novel bicyclic bromodomain inhibitors have *in vivo* antimyeloma activity in an athymic nude mouse strain of MM xenograft model using MM1.s cells	[186]
Mundy, G.R., Yoneda, T.	US20020022028	Methods of treating multiple myeloma and myeloma-induced bone resorption using integrin antagonists	Antagonists of 4 integri/alpha 4 integrin ligand adhesion are useful in suppressing bone destruction associated with MM	[187]

Abbreviations: MM - Multiple Myeloma

CURRENT & FUTURE DEVELOPMENTS

Multiple myeloma is an incurable condition that arises in the Bone Marrow (BM), and occasionally in extramedullary sites in the late clinical phase. It is the second most frequent hematological malignancy, accounting for 1% of all cancers and 13% of hematological malignancies. The introduction of novel drugs has allowed significant progress to be made in the treatment of MM over the past 15 years. Novel agents have prolonged survival and durable responses are now commonly observed. However, most patients eventually relapse, with the duration of response decreasing with each line of therapy, eventually showing multiple drug resistance. In particular, high-risk and relapsed/refractory patients remain challenging to treat and their outcome remains poor. In recent years, the appearance of several new drugs with different mechanisms of action has influenced the approach to treat both previously-untreated patients and those with relapsed/refractory disease. Novel agents include third-generation immunomodulatory drugs (pomalidomide), second-generation proteasome inhibitors (carfilzomib and ixazomib) and histone deacetylase inhibitors (panobinostat). Several other agents with various chemical structures and mechanisms of action have also been developed in recent years and show promising results in preclinical studies and early clinical trials. These include new proteasome inhibitors such as marizomib, ONX 0912 and MLN 9708, as well as kinase inhibitors of mTOR, HSP90 and new antibodies against CS-1, CD38, and IL-6. A range of other promising agents have also been developed, some key ones being the oral BCL-2 inhibitor venetoclax, an oral inhibitor of the nuclear export protein exportin 1 (XPO1) selinexor, the peptidase-potentiated alkylating drug melflufen, and the novel ATP-competitive inhibitor afursertib. Anti-PD1 and anti PDL1 checkpoint-inhibitors like pembrolizumab, nivolumab and durvolumab have also been evaluated with promising results in heavily-pretreated MM patients.

Although these agents can improve treatment efficacy in MM patients when used in combination with conventional drugs, further research is needed to gain a better understanding of the mechanisms of resistance to the drugs, including the pathways and proteins involved in these processes. In addition, cellular therapies, particularly those associated with Chimeric Antigen Receptor (CAR) T cells, have been regarded as promising strategies for treating B-cell lymphoid malignancies. In MM, B-Cell Maturation Antigen (BCMA) is a possible target for Chimeric Antigen Receptor (CAR)-transfected T cells (CAR T cells). Recently, CART-BCMA infusions, with or without lymphodepleting chemotherapy, have been shown to be clinically active in heavily-pretreated MM patients. Clinical trials based on CD38 CAR T cells in MM patients are currently ongoing (www.clinicaltrials.gov). Success in these studies should improve the outcomes of MM therapy by increasing the efficacy of available drugs and reducing their toxicity.

PATIENT CONSENT

Patient consent is not applicable in this chapter.

CONSENT FOR PUBLICATION

The authors guarantee that the contribution to the work has not been previously published elsewhere.

FUNDING

This work was supported in part by the NCN grant 2016/23/B/NZ5/02529. No writing assistance was utilized in the production of this chapter.

CONFLICT OF INTEREST

The authors confirm that this chapter content has no conflicts of interest.

ACKNOWLEDGEMENTS

We thank Edward Lowczowski and Anna Rychter from the Medical University of Lodz for editorial assistance.

REFERENCES

[1]   Hideshima T, Mitsiades C, Tonon G, Richardson PG, Anderson KC. Understanding multiple myeloma pathogenesis in the bone marrow to identify new therapeutic targets. Nat Rev Cancer 2007; 7(8): 585-98.
[http://dx.doi.org/10.1038/nrc2189] [PMID: 17646864]

[2]   Palumbo A, Anderson K. Multiple myeloma. N Engl J Med 2011; 364(11): 1046-60.
[http://dx.doi.org/10.1056/NEJMra1011442] [PMID: 21410373]

[3]   Becker N. Epidemiology of multiple myeloma. Recent Results Cancer Res 2011; 183: 25-35.
        [http://dx.doi.org/10.1007/978-3-540-85772-3_2] [PMID: 21509679]

[4]   Siegel RL, Miller KD, Jemal A. Cancer Statistics, 2017. CA Cancer J Clin 2017; 67(1): 7-30.
        [http://dx.doi.org/10.3322/caac.21387] [PMID: 28055103]

[5]   Ferlay J, Soerjomataram I, Dikshit R, *et al.* Cancer incidence and mortality worldwide: Sources,
        methods and major patterns in GLOBOCAN 2012. Int J Cancer 2015; 136(5): E359-86.
        [http://dx.doi.org/10.1002/ijc.29210] [PMID: 25220842]

[6]   Palumbo A, Bringhen S, Ludwig H, *et al.* Personalized therapy in multiple myeloma according to
        patient age and vulnerability: A report of the European Myeloma Network (EMN). Blood 2011;
        118(17): 4519-29.
        [http://dx.doi.org/10.1182/blood-2011-06-358812] [PMID: 21841166]

[7]   Moreau P, San Miguel J, Sonneveld P, *et al.* Multiple myeloma: ESMO Clinical Practice Guidelines
        for diagnosis, treatment and follow-up. Ann Oncol 2017; 28 (suppl_4): iv52-61.
        [http://dx.doi.org/10.1093/annonc/mdx096] [PMID: 28453614]

[8]   Criteria for the classification of monoclonal gammopathies, multiple myeloma and related disorders: A
        report of the International Myeloma Working Group. Br J Haematol 2003; 121(5): 749-57.
        [http://dx.doi.org/10.1046/j.1365-2141.2003.04355.x] [PMID: 12780789]

[9]   Kyle RA, Therneau TM, Rajkumar SV, *et al.* Prevalence of monoclonal gammopathy of undetermined
        significance. N Engl J Med 2006; 354(13): 1362-9.
        [http://dx.doi.org/10.1056/NEJMoa054494] [PMID: 16571879]

[10]   Kyle RA, Durie BG, Rajkumar SV, *et al.* Monoclonal gammopathy of undetermined significance
        (MGUS) and smoldering (asymptomatic) multiple myeloma: IMWG consensus perspectives risk
        factors for progression and guidelines for monitoring and management. Leukemia 2010; 24(6): 1121-
        7.
        [http://dx.doi.org/10.1038/leu.2010.60] [PMID: 20410922]

[11]   Landgren O, Kyle RA, Pfeiffer RM, *et al.* Monoclonal gammopathy of undetermined significance
        (MGUS) consistently precedes multiple myeloma: A prospective study. Blood 2009; 113(22): 5412-7.
        [http://dx.doi.org/10.1182/blood-2008-12-194241] [PMID: 19179464]

[12]   Weiss BM, Abadie J, Verma P, Howard RS, Kuehl WM. A monoclonal gammopathy precedes
        multiple myeloma in most patients. Blood 2009; 113(22): 5418-22.
        [http://dx.doi.org/10.1182/blood-2008-12-195008] [PMID: 19234139]

[13]   Rajkumar SV, Dimopoulos MA, Palumbo A, *et al.* International Myeloma Working Group updated
        criteria for the diagnosis of multiple myeloma. Lancet Oncol 2014; 15(12): e538-48.
        [http://dx.doi.org/10.1016/S1470-2045(14)70442-5] [PMID: 25439696]

[14]   Landgren O, Morgan GJ. Biologic frontiers in multiple myeloma: From biomarker identification to
        clinical practice. Clin Cancer Res 2014; 20(4): 804-13.
        [http://dx.doi.org/10.1158/1078-0432.CCR-13-2159] [PMID: 24270684]

[15]   Morgan GJ, Walker BA, Davies FE. The genetic architecture of multiple myeloma. Nat Rev Cancer
        2012; 12(5): 335-48.
        [http://dx.doi.org/10.1038/nrc3257] [PMID: 22495321]

[16]   Tibullo D, Di Rosa M, Giallongo C, *et al.* Bortezomib modulates CHIT1 and YKL40 in monocyte-
        derived osteoclast and in myeloma cells. Front Pharmacol 2015; 6: 226.
        [http://dx.doi.org/10.3389/fphar.2015.00226] [PMID: 26528182]

[17]   Wang J, De Veirman K, De Beule N, *et al.* The bone marrow microenvironment enhances multiple
        myeloma progression by exosome-mediated activation of myeloid-derived suppressor cells.
        Oncotarget 2015; 6(41): 43992-4004.
        [http://dx.doi.org/10.18632/oncotarget.6083] [PMID: 26556857]

[18]   Morgan GJ, Rasche L. Maintaining therapeutic progress in multiple myeloma by integrating genetic and biological advances into the clinic. Expert Rev Hematol 2018; 11(7): 513-23.
[http://dx.doi.org/10.1080/17474086.2018.1489718] [PMID: 29944024]

[19]   Mori Y, Shimizu N, Dallas M, *et al.* Anti-alpha4 integrin antibody suppresses the development of multiple myeloma and associated osteoclastic osteolysis. Blood 2004; 104(7): 2149-54.
[http://dx.doi.org/10.1182/blood-2004-01-0236] [PMID: 15138161]

[20]   Roy P, Sarkar UA, Basak S. The NF-κB activating pathways in multiple myeloma. Biomedicines 2018; 6(2): E59.
[http://dx.doi.org/10.3390/biomedicines6020059] [PMID: 29772694]

[21]   Vacca A, Ribatti D. Angiogenesis and vasculogenesis in multiple myeloma: Role of inflammatory cells. Recent Results Cancer Res 2011; 183: 87-95.
[http://dx.doi.org/10.1007/978-3-540-85772-3_4] [PMID: 21509681]

[22]   Hose D, Moreaux J, Meissner T, *et al.* Induction of angiogenesis by normal and malignant plasma cells. Blood 2009; 114(1): 128-43.
[http://dx.doi.org/10.1182/blood-2008-10-184226] [PMID: 19299335]

[23]   Vacca A, Ria R, Semeraro F, *et al.* Endothelial cells in the bone marrow of patients with multiple myeloma. Blood 2003; 102(9): 3340-8.
[http://dx.doi.org/10.1182/blood-2003-04-1338] [PMID: 12855563]

[24]   Terpos E, Ntanasis-Stathopoulos I, Dimopoulos MA. Myeloma bone disease: From biology findings to treatment approaches. Blood 2019; 133(14): 1534-9.
[http://dx.doi.org/10.1182/blood-2018-11-852459] [PMID: 30760454]

[25]   Giuliani N, Ferretti M, Bolzoni M, *et al.* Increased osteocyte death in multiple myeloma patients: Role in myeloma-induced osteoclast formation. Leukemia 2012; 26(6): 1391-401.
[http://dx.doi.org/10.1038/leu.2011.381] [PMID: 22289923]

[26]   Christoulas D, Terpos E, Dimopoulos MA. Pathogenesis and management of myeloma bone disease. Expert Rev Hematol 2009; 2(4): 385-98.
[http://dx.doi.org/10.1586/ehm.09.36] [PMID: 21082944]

[27]   Merico F, Bergui L, Gregoretti MG, *et al.* Cytokines involved in the progression of multiple myeloma. Clin Exp Immunol 1993; 92(1): 27-31.
[http://dx.doi.org/10.1111/j.1365-2249.1993.tb05943.x] [PMID: 8467562]

[28]   Komander D, Clague MJ, Urbé S. Breaking the chains: Structure and function of the deubiquitinases. Nat Rev Mol Cell Biol 2009; 10(8): 550-63.
[http://dx.doi.org/10.1038/nrm2731] [PMID: 19626045]

[29]   Kumar SK, Dispenzieri A, Lacy MQ, *et al.* Continued improvement in survival in multiple myeloma: Changes in early mortality and outcomes in older patients. Leukemia 2014; 28(5): 1122-8.
[http://dx.doi.org/10.1038/leu.2013.313] [PMID: 24157580]

[30]   Hideshima T, Mitsiades C, Akiyama M, *et al.* Molecular mechanisms mediating antimyeloma activity of proteasome inhibitor PS-341. Blood 2003; 101(4): 1530-4.
[http://dx.doi.org/10.1182/blood-2002-08-2543] [PMID: 12393500]

[31]   Obeng EA, Carlson LM, Gutman DM, Harrington WJ Jr, Lee KP, Boise LH. Proteasome inhibitors induce a terminal unfolded protein response in multiple myeloma cells. Blood 2006; 107(12): 4907-16.
[http://dx.doi.org/10.1182/blood-2005-08-3531] [PMID: 16507771]

[32]   Mitsiades N, Mitsiades CS, Poulaki V, *et al.* Molecular sequelae of proteasome inhibition in human multiple myeloma cells. Proc Natl Acad Sci USA 2002; 99(22): 14374-9.
[http://dx.doi.org/10.1073/pnas.202445099] [PMID: 12391322]

[33]   Yarde DN, Oliveira V, Mathews L, *et al.* Targeting the Fanconi anemia/BRCA pathway circumvents drug resistance in multiple myeloma. Cancer Res 2009; 69(24): 9367-75.

[http://dx.doi.org/10.1158/0008-5472.CAN-09-2616] [PMID: 19934314]

[34] Teicher BA, Tomaszewski JE. Proteasome inhibitors. Biochem Pharmacol 2015; 96(1): 1-9.
      [http://dx.doi.org/10.1016/j.bcp.2015.04.008] [PMID: 25935605]

[35] Boccadoro M, Morgan G, Cavenagh J. Preclinical evaluation of the proteasome inhibitor bortezomib
      in cancer therapy. Cancer Cell Int 2005; 5(1): 18.
      [http://dx.doi.org/10.1186/1475-2867-5-18] [PMID: 15929791]

[36] Meusser B, Hirsch C, Jarosch E, Sommer T. ERAD: The long road to destruction. Nat Cell Biol 2005;
      7(8): 766-72.
      [http://dx.doi.org/10.1038/ncb0805-766] [PMID: 16056268]

[37] Voorhees PM, Orlowski RZ. The proteasome and proteasome inhibitors in cancer therapy. Annu Rev
      Pharmacol Toxicol 2006; 46: 189-213.
      [http://dx.doi.org/10.1146/annurev.pharmtox.46.120604.141300] [PMID: 16402903]

[38] Adams J, Palombella VJ, Sausville EA, *et al.* Proteasome inhibitors: A novel class of potent and
      effective antitumor agents. Cancer Res 1999; 59(11): 2615-22.
      [PMID: 10363983]

[39] Teicher BA, Ara G, Herbst R, Palombella VJ, Adams J. The proteasome inhibitor PS-341 in cancer
      therapy. Clin Cancer Res 1999; 5(9): 2638-45.
      [PMID: 10499643]

[40] Mohan M, Matin A, Davies FE. Update on the optimal use of bortezomib in the treatment of multiple
      myeloma. Cancer Manag Res 2017; 9: 51-63.
      [http://dx.doi.org/10.2147/CMAR.S105163] [PMID: 28280389]

[41] Kane RC, Bross PF, Farrell AT, Pazdur R. Velcade: U.S. FDA approval for the treatment of multiple
      myeloma progressing on prior therapy. Oncologist 2003; 8(6): 508-13.
      [http://dx.doi.org/10.1634/theoncologist.8-6-508] [PMID: 14657528]

[42] Kane RC, Farrell AT, Sridhara R, Pazdur R. United States Food and Drug Administration approval
      summary: Bortezomib for the treatment of progressive multiple myeloma after one prior therapy. Clin
      Cancer Res 2006; 12(10): 2955-60.
      [http://dx.doi.org/10.1158/1078-0432.CCR-06-0170] [PMID: 16707588]

[43] Raedler L. Velcade (Bortezomib) receives 2 new FDA indications: For retreatment of patients with
      multiple myeloma and for first-line treatment of patients with mantle-cell lymphoma. Am Health Drug
      Benefits 2015; 8: 135-40.
      [PMID: 26629279]

[44] Moreau P, Pylypenko H, Grosicki S, *et al.* Subcutaneous versus intravenous administration of
      bortezomib in patients with relapsed multiple myeloma: A randomised, Phase 3, non-inferiority study.
      Lancet Oncol 2011; 12(5): 431-40.
      [http://dx.doi.org/10.1016/S1470-2045(11)70081-X] [PMID: 21507715]

[45] Leal TB, Remick SC, Takimoto CH, *et al.* Dose-escalating and pharmacological study of bortezomib
      in adult cancer patients with impaired renal function: A National Cancer Institute Organ Dysfunction
      Working Group Study. Cancer Chemother Pharmacol 2011; 68(6): 1439-47.
      [http://dx.doi.org/10.1007/s00280-011-1637-5] [PMID: 21479634]

[46] LoRusso PM, Venkatakrishnan K, Ramanathan RK, *et al.* Pharmacokinetics and safety of bortezomib
      in patients with advanced malignancies and varying degrees of liver dysfunction: Phase I NCI Organ
      Dysfunction Working Group Study NCI-6432. Clin Cancer Res 2012; 18(10): 2954-63.
      [http://dx.doi.org/10.1158/1078-0432.CCR-11-2873] [PMID: 22394984]

[47] Hill A, Redd C, Gotham D, Erbacher I, Meldrum J, Harada R. Estimated generic prices of cancer
      medicines deemed cost-ineffective in England: A cost estimation analysis. BMJ Open 2017; 7(1):
      e011965.
      [http://dx.doi.org/10.1136/bmjopen-2016-011965] [PMID: 28110283]

[48] Rajkumar SV. Multiple myeloma: 2016 update on diagnosis, risk-stratification, and management. Am J Hematol 2016; 91(7): 719-34.
[http://dx.doi.org/10.1002/ajh.24402] [PMID: 27291302]

[49] Dimopoulos MA, Roussou M, Gavriatopoulou M, *et al.* Outcomes of newly diagnosed myeloma patients requiring dialysis: Renal recovery, importance of rapid response and survival benefit. Blood Cancer J 2017; 7(6): e571.
[http://dx.doi.org/10.1038/bcj.2017.49] [PMID: 28622304]

[50] Kumar SK, Callander NS, Alsina M, *et al.* Multiple Myeloma, Version 3.2017, NCCN Clinical Practice Guidelines in Oncology. J Natl Compr Canc Netw 2017; 15(2): 230-69.
[http://dx.doi.org/10.6004/jnccn.2017.0023] [PMID: 28188192]

[51] Mai EK, Bertsch U, Dürig J, *et al.* Phase III trial of bortezomib, cyclophosphamide and dexamethasone (VCD) versus bortezomib, doxorubicin and dexamethasone (PAd) in newly diagnosed myeloma. Leukemia 2015; 29(8): 1721-9.
[http://dx.doi.org/10.1038/leu.2015.80] [PMID: 25787915]

[52] Mian M, Pescosta N, Badiali S, *et al.* Phase II trial to investigate efficacy and safety of bendamustine, dexamethasone and thalidomide in relapsed or refractory multiple myeloma patients after treatment with lenalidomide and bortezomib. Br J Haematol 2019; 185(5): 944-7.

[53] Fenk R, Michael M, Zohren F, *et al.* Escalation therapy with bortezomib, dexamethasone and bendamustine for patients with relapsed or refractory multiple myeloma. Leuk Lymphoma 2007; 48(12): 2345-51.
[http://dx.doi.org/10.1080/10428190701694194] [PMID: 18067009]

[54] Neben K, Lokhorst HM, Jauch A, *et al.* Administration of bortezomib before and after autologous stem cell transplantation improves outcome in multiple myeloma patients with deletion 17p. Blood 2012; 119(4): 940-8.
[http://dx.doi.org/10.1182/blood-2011-09-379164] [PMID: 22160383]

[55] Einsele H, Knop S, Vogel M, *et al.* Response-adapted consolidation with bortezomib after ASCT improves progression-free survival in newly diagnosed multiple myeloma. Leukemia 2017; 31(6): 1463-6.
[http://dx.doi.org/10.1038/leu.2017.83] [PMID: 28293022]

[56] Dimopoulos MA, Weisel K, Moreau P, *et al.* Pomalidomide + bortezomib + low-dose dexamethasone *vs* bortezomib + low-dose dexamethasone as second-line treatment in patients with lenalidomide-pretreated multiple myeloma: A subgroup analysis of the Phase 3 Optimismm trial. In: American Society of Hematology - 60th ASH Annual Meeting and Exposition; San Diego, USA. 2018.

[57] Siegel DS, Martin T, Wang M, *et al.* A Phase 2 study of single-agent carfilzomib (PX-171-003-A1) in patients with relapsed and refractory multiple myeloma. Blood 2012; 120(14): 2817-25.
[http://dx.doi.org/10.1182/blood-2012-05-425934] [PMID: 22833546]

[58] Stewart AK, Rajkumar SV, Dimopoulos MA, *et al.* Carfilzomib, lenalidomide, and dexamethasone for relapsed multiple myeloma. N Engl J Med 2015; 372(2): 142-52.
[http://dx.doi.org/10.1056/NEJMoa1411321] [PMID: 25482145]

[59] Dimopoulos MA, Moreau P, Palumbo A, *et al.* Carfilzomib and dexamethasone versus bortezomib and dexamethasone for patients with relapsed or refractory multiple myeloma (ENDEAVOR): A randomised, Phase 3, open-label, multicentre study. Lancet Oncol 2016; 17(1): 27-38.
[http://dx.doi.org/10.1016/S1470-2045(15)00464-7] [PMID: 26671818]

[60] Sonneveld P, Zweegman S, Cavo M, *et al.* Carfilzomib, pomalidomide and dexamethasone (KPd) in patients with multiple myeloma refractory to bortezomib and lenalidomide. In: The EMN011 trial. American Society of Hematology - 60th ASH Annual Meeting and Exposition; San Diego, USA. 2018.

[61] Touzeau C, Moreau P. Ixazomib in the management of relapsed multiple myeloma. Future Oncol 2018; 14(20): 2013-20.

[http://dx.doi.org/10.2217/fon-2017-0710] [PMID: 29469592]

[62]   Langston M, Mazaik D, Elliott E, Peterson A, Andres P, Teng J. Novel crystalline form of a proteasome inhibitor. US20180044356, 2018.

[63]   Moreau P, Masszi T, Grzasko N, *et al.* Oral ixazomib, lenalidomide, and dexamethasone for multiple myeloma. N Engl J Med 2016; 374(17): 1621-34.
[http://dx.doi.org/10.1056/NEJMoa1516282] [PMID: 27119237]

[64]   Levin N, Spencer A, Harrison SJ, *et al.* Marizomib irreversibly inhibits proteasome to overcome compensatory hyperactivation in multiple myeloma and solid tumour patients. Br J Haematol 2016; 174(5): 711-20.
[http://dx.doi.org/10.1111/bjh.14113] [PMID: 27161872]

[65]   Richardson PG, Zimmerman TM, Hofmeister CC, *et al.* Phase 1 study of marizomib in relapsed or relapsed and refractory multiple myeloma: NPI-0052-101 Part 1. Blood 2016; 127(22): 2693-700.
[http://dx.doi.org/10.1182/blood-2015-12-686378] [PMID: 27009059]

[66]   Trikha M, Levin N, Winograd B. Use of a proteasome inhibitor for the treatment of central nervous system (CNS) cancers. WO2018169740, 2018.

[67]   Spencer A, Spencer A, Badros A, Laubach J, Harrison S, Zonder J, *et al.* Phase 1, multicenter, open-label, dose-escalation, combination study (NCT02103335) of pomalidomide (POM), marizomib (MRZ, NPI-0052), and dexamethasone (DEX) in patients with relapsed and refractory multiple myeloma (MM); study NPI-0052-107 preliminary results. In: International Myeloma Society - 17th International Myeloma Workshop; Roma, Italy. 2015.

[68]   Vij R, Savona M, Siegel DS, *et al.* Clinical profile of single-agent oprozomib in patients (Pts) with multiple myeloma (MM): Updated results from a multicenter, open-label, dose escalation Phase 1b/2 study. In: American Society of Hematology - 56th ASH Annual Meeting; San Francisco, USA. 2014.

[69]   Hari PN, Shain KH, Voorhees PM, *et al.* Oprozomib and dexamethasone in patients with relapsed and/or refractory multiple myeloma: Initial results from the dose escalation portion of a Phase 1b/2, multicenter, open-label study. In: American Society of Hematology - 56th ASH Annual Meeting; San Francisco, USA. 2014.

[70]   Shah J, Niesvizky R, Stadtmauer E, *et al.* Oprozomib, pomalidomide, and dexamethasone (OPomd) in patients (Pts) with relapsed and/or refractory multiple myeloma (RRMM): Initial results of a Phase 1b study (NCT01999335). In: American Society of Hematology - 57th ASH Annual Meeting and Exposition; Orlando, USA. 2015.

[71]   Vogl DT, Martin TG, Vij R, *et al.* Phase I/II study of the novel proteasome inhibitor delanzomib (CEP-18770) for relapsed and refractory multiple myeloma. Leuk Lymphoma 2017; 58(8): 1872-9.
[http://dx.doi.org/10.1080/10428194.2016.1263842] [PMID: 28140719]

[72]   Gozzetti A, Papini G, Candi V, Brambilla CZ, Sirianni S, Bocchia M. Second generation proteasome inhibitors in multiple myeloma. Anticancer Agents Med Chem 2017; 17(7): 920-6.
[http://dx.doi.org/10.2174/1871520616666160902101622] [PMID: 27592543]

[73]   Chang Y-N. Novel spiro and cyclic bis-benzylidine proteasome inhibitor for the treatment of cancer, diabetes and neurological disorders. WO2018140907, 2018.

[74]   Chiriva-Internati M, Figueroa JA, Cobos E. Galectin-3 inhibitor (GAL-3M) is associated with additive anti-myeloma and anti-solid tumor effects, decreased osteoclastogenesis and organ protection when used in combination with proteasome inhibitors. US201502169319, 2015.

[75]   Thibaudeau TA, Smith DM. A practical review of proteasome pharmacology. Pharmacol Rev 2019; 71(2): 170-97.
[http://dx.doi.org/10.1124/pr.117.015370] [PMID: 30867233]

[76]   Gaczynska ME, Osmulski PA. Rapapmycin analogs targeting proteasome function in the treatment of cancer. US9918968, 2018.

[77]   Farag Sherif S. Combined use of bendamustine, doxorubicin and bortezomib for the treatment of multiple myeloma. US20110217258, 2011.

[78]   Reboud-Ravaux M, Bernard E, Papapostolou D, Vanderesse R. Novel proteasome modulators. US20080076718, 2008.

[79]   Sanderson RD, Ramani VPC, Noseda A, Barbieri P. Roneparstat combined therapy of multiple myeloma. US20180050061, 2018.

[80]   Johnson RG Jr, Hannah AL, Cropp GF, Zhou YQ, Sherrill MJ. Method of treating multiple myeloma using 17-AAG or 17-Ag or a prodrug of either in combination with a proteasome inhibitor. WO2006119032, 2006.

[81]   Kunacheewa C, Orlowski RZ. New drugs in multiple myeloma. Annu Rev Med 2019; 70: 521-47.
[http://dx.doi.org/10.1146/annurev-med-112017-091045] [PMID: 30691369]

[82]   Szalat R, Munshi NC. Novel agents in multiple myeloma. Cancer J 2019; 25(1): 45-53.
[http://dx.doi.org/10.1097/PPO.0000000000000355] [PMID: 30694859]

[83]   Dimopoulos MA, Richardson PG, Moreau P, Anderson KC. Current treatment landscape for relapsed and/or refractory multiple myeloma. Nat Rev Clin Oncol 2015; 12(1): 42-54.
[http://dx.doi.org/10.1038/nrclinonc.2014.200] [PMID: 25421279]

[84]   Davies FE, Raje N, Hideshima T, *et al.* Thalidomide and immunomodulatory derivatives augment natural killer cell cytotoxicity in multiple myeloma. Blood 2001; 98(1): 210-6.
[http://dx.doi.org/10.1182/blood.V98.1.210] [PMID: 11418482]

[85]   Payvandi F, Wu L, Haley M, *et al.* Immunomodulatory drugs inhibit expression of cyclooxygenase-2 from TNF-alpha, IL-1beta, and LPS-stimulated human PBMC in a partially IL-10-dependent manner. Cell Immunol 2004; 230(2): 81-8.
[http://dx.doi.org/10.1016/j.cellimm.2004.09.003] [PMID: 15598423]

[86]   Vallet S, Palumbo A, Raje N, Boccadoro M, Anderson KC. Thalidomide and lenalidomide: Mechanism-based potential drug combinations. Leuk Lymphoma 2008; 49(7): 1238-45.
[http://dx.doi.org/10.1080/10428190802005191] [PMID: 18452080]

[87]   Chamberlain PP, Lopez-Girona A, Miller K, *et al.* Structure of the human Cereblon-DDB--lenalidomide complex reveals basis for responsiveness to thalidomide analogs. Nat Struct Mol Biol 2014; 21(9): 803-9.
[http://dx.doi.org/10.1038/nsmb.2874] [PMID: 25108355]

[88]   Azima H, Arthurs D. Control study of thalidomide (kevadon), a new hypnotic agent. Am J Psychiatry 1961; 118: 554-5.
[http://dx.doi.org/10.1176/ajp.118.6.554] [PMID: 13863556]

[89]   Somers GS. Thalidomide and congenital abnormalities. Lancet 1962; 1(7235): 912-3.
[http://dx.doi.org/10.1016/S0140-6736(62)91943-8] [PMID: 13915092]

[90]   Singhal S, Mehta J, Desikan R, *et al.* Antitumor activity of thalidomide in refractory multiple myeloma. N Engl J Med 1999; 341(21): 1565-71.
[http://dx.doi.org/10.1056/NEJM199911183412102] [PMID: 10564685]

[91]   Lara Ochoa JM. Use of thalidomide to inhibit the osteoclast-activation process associated with multiple myeloma disease. WO2010008263, 2010.

[92]   Dimopoulos M, Spencer A, Attal M, *et al.* Lenalidomide plus dexamethasone for relapsed or refractory multiple myeloma. N Engl J Med 2007; 357(21): 2123-32.
[http://dx.doi.org/10.1056/NEJMoa070594] [PMID: 18032762]

[93]   Weber DM, Chen C, Niesvizky R, *et al.* Lenalidomide plus dexamethasone for relapsed multiple myeloma in North America. N Engl J Med 2007; 357(21): 2133-42.
[http://dx.doi.org/10.1056/NEJMoa070596] [PMID: 18032763]

[94]   Holstein SA, Suman VJ, McCarthy PL. Update on the role of lenalidomide in patients with multiple myeloma. Ther Adv Hematol 2018; 9(7): 175-90.
[http://dx.doi.org/10.1177/2040620718775629] [PMID: 30013765]

[95]   O'Donnell EK, Laubach JP, Yee AJ, *et al.* A Phase II study of modified lenalidomide, bortezomib, and dexamethasone (RVD-lite) for transplant-ineligible patients with newly diagnosed multiple myeloma. In: American Society of Hematology - 57th ASH Annual Meeting and Exposition; Orlando, USA. 2015.

[96]   Hanaizi Z, Flores B, Hemmings R, *et al.* The European medicines agency review of pomalidomide in combination with low-dose dexamethasone for the treatment of adult patients with multiple myeloma: Summary of the scientific assessment of the committee for medicinal products for human use. Oncologist 2015; 20(3): 329-34.
[http://dx.doi.org/10.1634/theoncologist.2014-0073] [PMID: 25673103]

[97]   Miguel JS, Weisel K, Moreau P, *et al.* Pomalidomide plus low-dose dexamethasone versus high-dose dexamethasone alone for patients with relapsed and refractory multiple myeloma (MM-003): A randomised, open-label, Phase 3 trial. Lancet Oncol 2013; 14(11): 1055-66.
[http://dx.doi.org/10.1016/S1470-2045(13)70380-2] [PMID: 24007748]

[98]   Richardson PG, Rocafiguera AO, Beksac M, *et al.* Pomalidomide (POM), bortezomib, and low dose dexamethasone (PVd) *vs* bortezomib and low-dose dexamethasone (Vd) in lenalidomide (LEN)-exposed patients (pts) with relapsed or refractory multiple myeloma (RRMM): Phase 3 OPTIMISMM trial. 2018 American Society of Clinical Oncology (ASCO Annual meeting. Chicago, USA. 2018.

[99]   Ntanasis-Stathopoulos I, Terpos E, Dimopoulos MA. Optimizing immunomodulatory drug with proteasome inhibitor combinations in newly diagnosed multiple myeloma. Cancer J 2019; 25(1): 2-10.
[http://dx.doi.org/10.1097/PPO.0000000000000348] [PMID: 30694854]

[100]   Quayle SN, Jones SS. Combinations of histone deacetylase inhibitors and immunomodulatory drugs. US9949972, 2018.

[101]   Harada T, Hideshima T, Anderson KC. Histone deacetylase inhibitors in multiple myeloma: From bench to bedside. Int J Hematol 2016; 104(3): 300-9.
[http://dx.doi.org/10.1007/s12185-016-2008-0] [PMID: 27099225]

[102]   Chhabra S. Novel proteasome inhibitors and histone deacetylase inhibitors: Progress in myeloma therapeutics. Pharmaceuticals (Basel) 2017; 10(2)E40.
[http://dx.doi.org/10.3390/ph10020040] [PMID: 28398261]

[103]   Bradner JE, West N, Grachan ML, *et al.* Chemical phylogenetics of histone deacetylases. Nat Chem Biol 2010; 6(3): 238-43.
[http://dx.doi.org/10.1038/nchembio.313] [PMID: 20139990]

[104]   Dimopoulos M, Siegel DS, Lonial S, *et al.* Vorinostat or placebo in combination with bortezomib in patients with multiple myeloma (VANTAGE 088): A multicentre, randomised, double-blind study. Lancet Oncol 2013; 14(11): 1129-40.
[http://dx.doi.org/10.1016/S1470-2045(13)70398-X] [PMID: 24055414]

[105]   Waldschmidt JM, Keller A, Ihorst G, *et al.* Safety and efficacy of vorinostat, bortezomib, doxorubicin and dexamethasone in a Phase I/II study for relapsed or refractory multiple myeloma (VERUMM study: Vorinostat in elderly, relapsed and unfit multiple myeloma). Haematologica 2018; 103(10): e473-9.
[http://dx.doi.org/10.3324/haematol.2018.189969] [PMID: 29674494]

[106]   Sanchez L, Vesole DH, Richter JR, *et al.* A Phase IIb trial of vorinostat in combination with lenalidomide and dexamethasone in patients with multiple myeloma refractory to previous lenalidomide-containing regimens. Br J Haematol 2017; 176(3): 440-7.
[http://dx.doi.org/10.1111/bjh.14429] [PMID: 27859001]

[107]   Wolf JL, Siegel D, Goldschmidt H, *et al.* Phase II trial of the pan-deacetylase inhibitor panobinostat as

a single agent in advanced relapsed/refractory multiple myeloma. Leuk Lymphoma 2012; 53(9): 1820-3.
[http://dx.doi.org/10.3109/10428194.2012.661175] [PMID: 22288662]

[108] San-Miguel JF, Richardson PG, Günther A, *et al.* Phase Ib study of panobinostat and bortezomib in relapsed or relapsed and refractory multiple myeloma. J Clin Oncol 2013; 31(29): 3696-703.
[http://dx.doi.org/10.1200/JCO.2012.46.7068] [PMID: 24019544]

[109] Tzogani K, Hennik PV, Walsh I, *et al.* EMA review of panobinostat (Farydak) for the treatment of adult patients with relapsed and/or refractory multiple myeloma. Oncologist 2018; 23(7): 870.
[http://dx.doi.org/10.1634/theoncologist.2017-0301erratum] [PMID: 30037941]

[110] San-Miguel JF, Hungria VT, Yoon SS, *et al.* Panobinostat plus bortezomib and dexamethasone versus placebo plus bortezomib and dexamethasone in patients with relapsed or relapsed and refractory multiple myeloma: A multicentre, randomised, double-blind Phase 3 trial. Lancet Oncol 2014; 15(11): 1195-206.
[http://dx.doi.org/10.1016/S1470-2045(14)70440-1] [PMID: 25242045]

[111] Richardson PG, Hungria VT, Yoon SS, *et al.* Panobinostat plus bortezomib and dexamethasone in previously treated multiple myeloma: Outcomes by prior treatment. Blood 2016; 127(6): 713-21.
[http://dx.doi.org/10.1182/blood-2015-09-665018] [PMID: 26631116]

[112] San-Miguel JF, Hungria VT, Yoon SS, *et al.* Overall survival of patients with relapsed multiple myeloma treated with panobinostat or placebo plus bortezomib and dexamethasone (the PANORAMA 1 trial): A randomised, placebo-controlled, Phase 3 trial. Lancet Haematol 2016; 3(11): e506-15.
[http://dx.doi.org/10.1016/S2352-3026(16)30147-8] [PMID: 27751707]

[113] Popat R, Brown SR, Flanagan L, *et al.* Bortezomib, thalidomide, dexamethasone, and panobinostat for patients with relapsed multiple myeloma (MUK-six): A multicentre, open-label, Phase 1/2 trial. Lancet Haematol 2016; 3(12): e572-80.
[http://dx.doi.org/10.1016/S2352-3026(16)30165-X] [PMID: 27843120]

[114] Vogl DT, Raje N, Jagannath S, *et al.* Ricolinostat, the first selective histone deacetylase 6 inhibitor, in combination with bortezomib and dexamethasone for relapsed or refractory multiple myeloma. Clin Cancer Res 2017; 23(13): 3307-15.
[http://dx.doi.org/10.1158/1078-0432.CCR-16-2526] [PMID: 28053023]

[115] Mishima Y, Santo L, Eda H, *et al.* Ricolinostat (ACY-1215) induced inhibition of aggresome formation accelerates carfilzomib-induced multiple myeloma cell death. Br J Haematol 2015; 169(3): 423-34.
[http://dx.doi.org/10.1111/bjh.13315] [PMID: 25709080]

[116] Yee AJ, Bensinger WI, Supko JG, *et al.* Ricolinostat plus lenalidomide, and dexamethasone in relapsed or refractory multiple myeloma: A multicentre Phase 1b trial. Lancet Oncol 2016; 17(11): 1569-78.
[http://dx.doi.org/10.1016/S1470-2045(16)30375-8] [PMID: 27646843]

[117] North BJ, Almeciga-Pinto I, Tamang D, Yang M, Jones SS, Quayle SN. Enhancement of pomalidomide anti-tumor response with ACY-241, a selective HDAC6 inhibitor. PLoS One 2017; 12(3): e0173507.
[http://dx.doi.org/10.1371/journal.pone.0173507] [PMID: 28264055]

[118] Lichenstein H, Jeffers M, Qian X, Sehested M, Peterson KD, Ritchie J. Combination therapies using HDAC inhibitors. US20150231096, 2015.

[119] Lichenstein H, Edwards N, Ritchie J, Erichsen KD, Plumb J. deacetylaze(hdac) inhibitors for the treatment of cancer. US20180271852, 2018.

[120] Moreaux J, Klein B. Methods for predicting multiple myeloma treatment response. US20150275305, 2015.

[121] Stuttleworth SJ, Tomassi CD, Cecil ARL, Maccormick S, Nodes WJ, Silva FA. Novel histone

deacetylase inhibitors. US20180170876, 2018.

[122]   de Weers M, Tai YT, van der Veer MS, *et al.* Daratumumab, a novel therapeutic human CD38 monoclonal antibody, induces killing of multiple myeloma and other hematological tumors. J Immunol 2011; 186(3): 1840-8.
[http://dx.doi.org/10.4049/jimmunol.1003032] [PMID: 21187443]

[123]   Overdijk MB, Verploegen S, Bögels M, *et al.* Antibody-mediated phagocytosis contributes to the anti-tumor activity of the therapeutic antibody daratumumab in lymphoma and multiple myeloma. MAbs 2015; 7(2): 311-21.
[http://dx.doi.org/10.1080/19420862.2015.1007813] [PMID: 25760767]

[124]   Overdijk MB, Jansen JH, Nederend M, *et al.* The therapeutic CD38 monoclonal antibody daratumumab induces programmed cell death via Fc gamma receptor-mediated cross-linking. J Immunol 2016; 197(3): 807-13.
[http://dx.doi.org/10.4049/jimmunol.1501351] [PMID: 27316683]

[125]   Deaglio S, Mallone R, Baj G, *et al.* CD38/CD31, a receptor/ligand system ruling adhesion and signaling in human leukocytes. Chem Immunol 2000; 75: 99-120.
[http://dx.doi.org/10.1159/000058765] [PMID: 10851781]

[126]   Lonial S, Weiss BM, Usmani SZ, *et al.* Daratumumab monotherapy in patients with treatment-refractory multiple myeloma (SIRIUS): An open-label, randomised, Phase 2 trial. Lancet 2016; 387(10027): 1551-60.
[http://dx.doi.org/10.1016/S0140-6736(15)01120-4] [PMID: 26778538]

[127]   Lokhorst HM, Plesner T, Laubach JP, *et al.* Targeting CD38 with daratumumab monotherapy in multiple myeloma. N Engl J Med 2015; 373(13): 1207-19.
[http://dx.doi.org/10.1056/NEJMoa1506348] [PMID: 26308596]

[128]   Palumbo A, Chanan-Khan A, Weisel K, *et al.* Daratumumab, bortezomib, and dexamethasone for multiple myeloma. N Engl J Med 2016; 375(8): 754-66.
[http://dx.doi.org/10.1056/NEJMoa1606038] [PMID: 27557302]

[129]   Dimopoulos MA, Oriol A, Nahi H, *et al.* Daratumumab, lenalidomide, and dexamethasone for multiple myeloma. N Engl J Med 2016; 375(14): 1319-31.
[http://dx.doi.org/10.1056/NEJMoa1607751] [PMID: 27705267]

[130]   Chari A, Suvannasankha A, Fay JW, *et al.* Daratumumab plus pomalidomide and dexamethasone in relapsed and/or refractory multiple myeloma. Blood 2017; 130(8): 974-81.
[http://dx.doi.org/10.1182/blood-2017-05-785246] [PMID: 28637662]

[131]   Mateos MV, Dimopoulos MA, Cavo M, *et al.* Daratumumab plus bortezomib, melphalan, and prednisone for untreated myeloma. N Engl J Med 2018; 378(6): 518-28.
[http://dx.doi.org/10.1056/NEJMoa1714678] [PMID: 29231133]

[132]   Chari A, Lonial S, Mark TM, *et al.* Results of an early access treatment protocol of daratumumab in United States patients with relapsed or refractory multiple myeloma. Cancer 2018; 124(22): 4342-9.
[http://dx.doi.org/10.1002/cncr.31706] [PMID: 30395359]

[133]   van de Donk NW, Janmaat ML, Mutis T, *et al.* Monoclonal antibodies targeting CD38 in hematological malignancies and beyond. Immunol Rev 2016; 270(1): 95-112.
[http://dx.doi.org/10.1111/imr.12389] [PMID: 26864107]

[134]   Martin T, Strickland S, Glenn M, *et al.* Phase I trial of isatuximab monotherapy in the treatment of refractory multiple myeloma. Blood Cancer J 2019; 9(4): 41.
[http://dx.doi.org/10.1038/s41408-019-0198-4] [PMID: 30926770]

[135]   Martin T, Baz R, Benson DM, *et al.* A Phase 1b study of isatuximab plus lenalidomide and dexamethasone for relapsed/refractory multiple myeloma. Blood 2017; 129(25): 3294-303.
[http://dx.doi.org/10.1182/blood-2016-09-740787] [PMID: 28483761]

[136]   Mikhael J, Richardson P, Usmani SZ, *et al.* A Phase Ib study of isatuximab plus

pomalidomide/dexamethasone in relapsed/refractory multiple myeloma. Blood 2019; 134(2): 123-33.

[137]   Tai YT, Dillon M, Song W, *et al.* Anti-CS1 humanized monoclonal antibody HuLuc63 inhibits myeloma cell adhesion and induces antibody-dependent cellular cytotoxicity in the bone marrow milieu. Blood 2008; 112(4): 1329-37.
[http://dx.doi.org/10.1182/blood-2007-08-107292] [PMID: 17906076]

[138]   Lonial S, Dimopoulos M, Palumbo A, *et al.* Elotuzumab therapy for relapsed or refractory multiple myeloma. N Engl J Med 2015; 373(7): 621-31.
[http://dx.doi.org/10.1056/NEJMoa1505654] [PMID: 26035255]

[139]   Ribrag V, Avigan DE, Martinelli G, *et al.* Pembrolizumab monotherapy for relapsed/refractory multiple myeloma. In: European Hematology Association - 23rd EHA Congress; Stockholm, Sweden. 2018.

[140]   Badros A, Hyjek E, Ma N, *et al.* Pembrolizumab, pomalidomide, and low-dose dexamethasone for relapsed/refractory multiple myeloma. Blood 2017; 130(10): 1189-97.
[http://dx.doi.org/10.1182/blood-2017-03-775122] [PMID: 28461396]

[141]   Usmani SZ, Schjesvold F, Rocafiguera AO, Karlin L, Rifkin RM, San-Miguel J. A Phase 3 randomized study of pembrolizumab (pembro) plus lenalidomide (len) and low-dose dexamethasone (Rd) versus Rd for newly diagnosed and treatment-naive multiple myeloma (MM): KEYNOTE-185. 2018 American Society of Clinical Oncology (ASCO Annual meeting. Chicago, USA. 2018.

[142]   Lesokhin AM, Ansell SM, Armand P, *et al.* Nivolumab in patients with relapsed or refractory hematologic malignancy: Preliminary results of a Phase Ib study. J Clin Oncol 2016; 34(23): 2698-704.
[http://dx.doi.org/10.1200/JCO.2015.65.9789] [PMID: 27269947]

[143]   Baverel P, Dubois V, Jin C, *et al.* Population pharmacokinetics of durvalumab and fixed dosing regimens in patients with advanced solid tumors. 53rd Annual Meeting. Chicago, USA. 2017.
[http://dx.doi.org/10.1200/JCO.2017.35.15_suppl.2566]

[144]   Afar D, Andersen KC, Tai Y-T. Combination therapies based on anti-CS1 antibodies for treating multiple myeloma. EP3115049, 2017.

[145]   DeWeers M, Graus Y, Oprins J, Parren P, Van De WJ, Van Vugt M. Antibodies against CD38 for treatment of multiple myeloma. EP3312196, 2018.

[146]   Nandabalan K, Sharma H, Sapra AK, Upmanyu S. Novel immunomodulatory therapeutic strategies targeting tumors in cancer. US20180134771, 2018.

[147]   Martin MP, Olesen SH, Georg GI, Schönbrunn E. Cyclin-dependent kinase inhibitor dinaciclib interacts with the acetyl-lysine recognition site of bromodomains. ACS Chem Biol 2013; 8(11): 2360-5.
[http://dx.doi.org/10.1021/cb4003283] [PMID: 24007471]

[148]   Tang H, Xu L, Liang X, Gao G. Low dose dinaciclib enhances doxorubicin-induced senescence in myeloma RPMI8226 cells by transformation of the p21 and p16 pathways. Oncol Lett 2018; 16(5): 6608-14.
[http://dx.doi.org/10.3892/ol.2018.9474] [PMID: 30405800]

[149]   Kumar SK, LaPlant B, Chng WJ, *et al.* Dinaciclib, a novel CDK inhibitor, demonstrates encouraging single-agent activity in patients with relapsed multiple myeloma. Blood 2015; 125(3): 443-8.
[http://dx.doi.org/10.1182/blood-2014-05-573741] [PMID: 25395429]

[150]   Blangy A, Lane HA, d'Hérin P, Harper M, Kress M, Nigg EA. Phosphorylation by p34cdc2 regulates spindle association of human Eg5, a kinesin-related motor essential for bipolar spindle formation in vivo. Cell 1995; 83(7): 1159-69.
[http://dx.doi.org/10.1016/0092-8674(95)90142-6] [PMID: 8548803]

[151]   Shah JJ, Kaufman JL, Zonder JA, *et al.* A Phase 1 and 2 study of Filanesib alone and in combination with low-dose dexamethasone in relapsed/refractory multiple myeloma. Cancer 2017; 123(23): 4617-

30.
[http://dx.doi.org/10.1002/cncr.30892] [PMID: 28817190]

[152] Hernández-García S, San-Segundo L, González-Méndez L, *et al.* The kinesin spindle protein inhibitor filanesib enhances the activity of pomalidomide and dexamethasone in multiple myeloma. Haematologica 2017; 102(12): 2113-24.
[http://dx.doi.org/10.3324/haematol.2017.168666] [PMID: 28860344]

[153] Tolcher AW, Patnaik A, Papadopoulos KP, *et al.* Phase I study of the MEK inhibitor trametinib in combination with the AKT inhibitor afuresertib in patients with solid tumors and multiple myeloma. Cancer Chemother Pharmacol 2015; 75(1): 183-9.
[http://dx.doi.org/10.1007/s00280-014-2615-5] [PMID: 25417902]

[154] Kinoshita S, Ri M, Kanamori T, *et al.* Potent antitumor effect of combination therapy with sub-optimal doses of Akt inhibitors and pomalidomide plus dexamethasone in multiple myeloma. Oncol Lett 2018; 15(6): 9450-6.
[http://dx.doi.org/10.3892/ol.2018.8501] [PMID: 29928335]

[155] Spencer A, Yoon SS, Harrison SJ, *et al.* The novel AKT inhibitor afuresertib shows favorable safety, pharmacokinetics, and clinical activity in multiple myeloma. Blood 2014; 124(14): 2190-5.
[http://dx.doi.org/10.1182/blood-2014-03-559963] [PMID: 25075128]

[156] Garcia PD, Langowski JL, Wang Y, *et al.* Pan-PIM kinase inhibition provides a novel therapy for treating hematologic cancers. Clin Cancer Res 2014; 20(7): 1834-45.
[http://dx.doi.org/10.1158/1078-0432.CCR-13-2062] [PMID: 24474669]

[157] Raab MS, Ocio EM, Thomas SK, Günther A, Goh Y-T, Lebovic D, *et al.* Phase 1 study update of the novel Pan-Pim kinase inhibitor LGH447 in patients with relapsed/ refractory multiple myeloma. In: American Society of Hematology - 56th Annual Meeting; San Francisco, USA. 2014.

[158] Touzeau C, Dousset C, Le Gouill S, *et al.* The Bcl-2 specific BH3 mimetic ABT-199: A promising targeted therapy for t(11;14) multiple myeloma. Leukemia 2014; 28(1): 210-2.
[http://dx.doi.org/10.1038/leu.2013.216] [PMID: 23860449]

[159] Moreau P, Chanan-Khan A, Roberts AW, *et al.* Promising efficacy and acceptable safety of venetoclax plus bortezomib and dexamethasone in relapsed/refractory MM. Blood 2017; 130(22): 2392-400.
[http://dx.doi.org/10.1182/blood-2017-06-788323] [PMID: 28847998]

[160] Rahbari KJ, Nosrati JD, Spektor TM, Berenson JR. Venetoclax in combination with bortezomib, dexamethasone, and daratumumab for multiple myeloma. Clin Lymphoma Myeloma Leuk 2018; 18(9): e339-43.
[http://dx.doi.org/10.1016/j.clml.2018.06.003] [PMID: 30033209]

[161] Gonsalves WI, Buadi FK, Kumar SK. Combination therapy incorporating Bcl-2 inhibition with Venetoclax for the treatment of refractory primary plasma cell leukemia with t (11;14). Eur J Haematol 2018; 100(2): 215-7.
[http://dx.doi.org/10.1111/ejh.12986] [PMID: 29064593]

[162] Vaxman I, Sidiqi H, Gertz M. Venetoclax for the treatment of multiple myeloma. Expert Rev Hematol 2018; 11(12): 915-20.
[http://dx.doi.org/10.1080/17474086.2018.1548931] [PMID: 30428277]

[163] Kumar S, Kaufman JL, Gasparetto C, *et al.* Efficacy of venetoclax as targeted therapy for relapsed/refractory t(11;14) multiple myeloma. Blood 2017; 130(22): 2401-9.
[http://dx.doi.org/10.1182/blood-2017-06-788786] [PMID: 29018077]

[164] Costa LJ, Stadtmauer EA, Morgan G, *et al.* Phase 2 study of venetoclax plus carfilzomib and dexamethasone in patients with relapsed/refractory multiple myeloma. American Society of Clinical Oncology (ASCO 54th Annual Meeting. Chicago, USA. 2018.

[165] Chauhan D, Ray A, Viktorsson K, *et al. In vitro* and *in vivo* antitumor activity of a novel alkylating agent, melphalan-flufenamide, against multiple myeloma cells. Clin Cancer Res 2013; 19(11): 3019-

31.
[http://dx.doi.org/10.1158/1078-0432.CCR-12-3752] [PMID: 23584492]

[166]   Ray A, Ravillah D, Das DS, *et al.* A novel alkylating agent Melflufen induces irreversible DNA damage and cytotoxicity in multiple myeloma cells. Br J Haematol 2016; 174(3): 397-409.
[http://dx.doi.org/10.1111/bjh.14065] [PMID: 27098276]

[167]   Wickström M, Nygren P, Larsson R, *et al.* Melflufen - a peptidase-potentiated alkylating agent in clinical trials. Oncotarget 2017; 8(39): 66641-55.
[http://dx.doi.org/10.18632/oncotarget.18420] [PMID: 29029544]

[168]   Richardson P, Ocio E, Oriol A, Larocca A, Rodriguez Otero P, Moreb J, *et al.* OP-106 Horizon - Melflufen therapy for RR MM patients refractory to daratumumab and/or pomalidomide; Updated results and first report on PFS. In: American Society of Hematology - 60th ASH Annual Meeting and Exposition; San Diego, USA. 2018.

[169]   Burki TK. Selinexor and dexamethasone in multiple myeloma. Lancet Oncol 2018; 19(3): e146.
[http://dx.doi.org/10.1016/S1470-2045(18)30089-5] [PMID: 29429914]

[170]   Chen C, Siegel D, Gutierrez M, *et al.* Safety and efficacy of selinexor in relapsed or refractory multiple myeloma and Waldenstrom macroglobulinemia. Blood 2018; 131(8): 855-63.
[http://dx.doi.org/10.1182/blood-2017-08-797886] [PMID: 29203585]

[171]   Vogl DT, Dingli D, Cornell RF, *et al.* Selective inhibition of nuclear export with oral selinexor for treatment of relapsed or refractory multiple myeloma. J Clin Oncol 2018; 36(9): 859-66.
[http://dx.doi.org/10.1200/JCO.2017.75.5207] [PMID: 29381435]

[172]   Chari A, Vogl DT, Dimopoulos MA, *et al.* Results of the pivotal STORM study (Part 2) in penta-refractory multiple myeloma (MM): Deep and durable responses with oral selinexor plus low dose dexamethasone in patients with penta-refractory MM. In: American Society of Hematology - 60th ASH Annual Meeting and Exposition; San Diego, USA. 2018.

[173]   Bahlis NJ, Sutherland H, White D, *et al.* Selinexor plus low-dose bortezomib and dexamethasone for patients with relapsed or refractory multiple myeloma. Blood 2018; 132(24): 2546-54.
[http://dx.doi.org/10.1182/blood-2018-06-858852] [PMID: 30352784]

[174]   Chen CI, Sutherland HJ, Kotb R, *et al.* Selinexor plus pomalidomide and low dose dexamethasone (SPd) in patients with relapsed or refractory multiple myeloma. In: American Society of Hematology - 60th ASH Annual Meeting and Exposition; San Diego, USA. 2018.

[175]   Pyne NJ, Pyne S. Sphingosine kinase 2 and multiple myeloma. Oncotarget 2017; 8(27): 43596-7.
[http://dx.doi.org/10.18632/oncotarget.17420]

[176]   Venkata JK, An N, Stuart R, *et al.* Inhibition of sphingosine kinase 2 downregulates the expression of c-Myc and Mcl-1 and induces apoptosis in multiple myeloma. Blood 2014; 124(12): 1915-25.
[http://dx.doi.org/10.1182/blood-2014-03-559385] [PMID: 25122609]

[177]   Sundaramoorthy P, Gasparetto C, Kang Y. The combination of a sphingosine kinase 2 inhibitor (ABC294640) and a Bcl-2 inhibitor (ABT-199) displays synergistic anti-myeloma effects in myeloma cells without a t(11;14) translocation. Cancer Med 2018. Epub ahead of Print
[http://dx.doi.org/10.1002/cam4.1543] [PMID: 29761903]

[178]   Yubin Kang Y, Fan S, Sundaramoorthy P, *et al.* Sphingosine kinase 2 (SK2) targeting in the treatment of multiple myeloma: Preclinical and Phase I studies of opaganib, an SK 2 inhibitor, in multiple myeloma. In: 30th EORTC-NCI-AACR Symposium; Dublin, Irland. 2018.

[179]   Chesi M, Fonseca R. Antibodies create killer bonds in myeloma. Cancer Cell 2017; 31(3): 305-7.
[http://dx.doi.org/10.1016/j.ccell.2017.02.011] [PMID: 28292432]

[180]   Hipp S, Tai YT, Blanset D, *et al.* A novel BCMA/CD3 bispecific T-cell engager for the treatment of multiple myeloma induces selective lysis *in vitro* and *in vivo*. Leukemia 2017; 31(8): 1743-51.
[http://dx.doi.org/10.1038/leu.2016.388] [PMID: 28025583]

[181] Topp MS, Duell J, Zugmaier G, *et al.* Treatment with AMG 420, an anti-B-cell maturation antigen (BCMA) bispecific T-cell engager (BiTE®) antibody construct, induces Minimal Residual Disease (MRD) negative complete responses in relapsed and/or refractory (R/R) Multiple Myeloma (MM) patients: Results of a First-In-Human (FIH) Phase I dose escalation study. In: American Society of Hematology - 60th ASH Annual Meeting and Exposition; San Diego, USA. 2018.

[182] MacKinnon AL, Rodriguez ML. Treatment of multiple myeloma with heterocyclic inhibitors of glutaminase. WO2016014890, 2016.

[183] Adams J. Carboline derivatives as inhibitors of IKB in the treatment of multiple myeloma and others cancers. WO2003039545, 2003.

[184] Deng J. Use of camptothecin derivative in preparing pharmaceutical used for treating multiple myeloma. EP3100734, 2016.

[185] Scholz A. Use of 4-(4-fluoro-2-methoxyphenyl)-N-{3-[(s-methylsulfonimidoyl) methyl]phenyl}-1,3,5-triazin-2-amine for treating multiple myeloma. US20180078560, 2018.

[186] Quinn, J.F., Duffy, B.C., Liu, S., Wang, R., Jiang, M.X., Martin, G.S., Wagner, G.S., Young, P.R. Novel bicyclic bromodomain inhibitors. US20180161337, 2018.

[187] Mundy, G.R., Yoneda, T. Methods of treating multiple myeloma and myeloma-induced bone resorption using integrin antagonists. US20020022028, 2002.

CHAPTER 2

Synthetic Estrogens Deregulate Estrogen Receptors Inducing Thromboembolic Complications and Cancer

Zsuzsanna Suba[*]

National Institute of Oncology Department of Molecular Pathology Address: H-1122, Ráth György Str. 7-9 Budapest, Hungary

Abstract: In the early 1940's, the US Food and Drug Administration (FDA) approved marketing of synthetic estrogens; non steroidal Diethylstilbestrol (DES) and Ethinylestradiol (EE) as well as Conjugated Equine Estrogens (CEEs) for medical purposes. High Dose Estrogen (HDE) therapy using DES and EE was introduced into the treatment of advanced breast cancer in postmenopausal women. Oral contraceptives (OCs) comprising EE were developed in the early 1960s and EE became a standard component of near all combined forms of contraceptive pills. Use of exclusively synthetic estrogens for both HDE therapy of breast cancer and contraception ensured a possibility for clear evaluations of the risks and benefits of synthetic hormone use. HDE therapy for breast cancer induced serious toxicity affecting near all organs, suggesting a genome-wide disturbance in cellular mechanisms. OCs comprising low doses of EE which may induce arterial and venous thromboembolic events and show ambiguous correlations with cancer risk at different sites by means of altered regulation of Estrogen Receptors (ERs). In contrast, for menopausal Hormone Replacement Therapy (HRT) both synthetic and natural estrogens extracted from biological samples were prescribed. Among postmenopausal women, the use of estrogens with different origin and even their combinations with synthetic progestins resulted in a chaos of quite controversial clinical experiences concerning the risks for arterial and venous thromboembolism and for cancers of breasts and endometrium. Analysis of the effects of specific HRT types in postmenopausal women justified that horse urine derived CEE without synthetic progestin is a highly beneficial formula against breast cancer, coronary heart disease and bone loss. The presented study reveals that an 80 year period of synthetic hormone prescription may be blamed for the misbelief that ERs exposed to elevated endogenous estrogen concentrations may be deregulated and drive cancer promoting changes. In tumors constitutively upregulating ER alpha expression, recent patents disclose amplifying *ESR1* mutations.

Keywords: Antiestrogen, aromatase inhibitor, cancer treatment, estrogen rec-

---

[*] **Corresponding author Zsuzsanna Suba:** National Institute of Oncology Department of Molecular Pathology Address: H-1122, Ráth György Str. 7-9 Budapest, Hungary; Tel: 00 36 1 224 86 00; Fax: 00 36 1 224 86 20; E-mail: subazdr@gmail.com

Atta-ur-Rahman and Khurshid Zaman (Eds.)

eptor, estrogen paradox, ethinylestradiol, genomic stability, growth factor receptor, high dose estrogen therapy, hormone replacement therapy, oral contraceptives, synthetic estrogen, tamoxifen, tumor response.

1. INTRODUCTION

The paradoxical effects of ovarian hormones on both the promotion and prevention of breast cancer have been debated for over 80 years.

In 1896, a regression of breast cancer was achieved by estrogen hormone withdrawal via ovariectomy in premenopausal patients [1]. From that time onwards, hypoestrogenism as an anticancer means gained great popularity in medical practice and defined the unique pathway of breast cancer care until today [2]. In reality, living organisms are dynamic, self regulating systems. In women, an abrupt withdrawal of the crucial estrogen hormone induces compensatory mechanisms via an abundant estrogen synthesis at peripheral sites accidentally leading to transient tumor regression [3].

In the early 1940s, the US Food and Drug Administration (FDA) approved the marketing of synthetic estrogens; non steroidal Diethylstilbestrol (DES) and Ethinylestradiol (EE) as well as Conjugated Equine Estrogens (CEEs) for medical practice [4].

High Dose Estrogen (HDE) therapy using DES and EE was introduced into the treatment of advanced breast cancer in postmenopausal women from 1943 onward [5, 6]. In contrast, CEEs have not been investigated for the treatment of breast cancer, because the mixture of horse urine derived estrogens seemed to be dangerous attributed to its unknown toxicity at higher doses [7]. The use of exclusively synthetic estrogens against breast cancer as a HDE therapy ensured a possibility for the clear evaluation of risks and benefits of synthetic hormones in high doses.

In patients treated with HDE, all toxic side effects, including cardiovascular and gastrointestinal toxicity were regarded as unavoidable complications of estrogen treatment apparently similar to those found in correlation with high endogenous estrogen levels [7]. Nevertheless, during healthy pregnancy, endogenous 17-beta estradiol level in the serum increases exponentially up to a 300 fold elevation at term and there are no toxic complications [8].

In breast cancer cases treated with synthetic estrogens in high doses, in addition to modest regression rates (< 30%) of tumors, the experienced serious toxic effects suggest a genome wide alteration of cellular mechanisms instead of strong agonistic activation of Estrogen Receptors (ERs) [9]. Today, the recurrence of breast cancer and a fatal outcome of the disease are not predictable even in case of tumors diagnosed and treated at the earliest stage, justifying that our standard approach to breast cancer therapy is not appropriate [2].

Oral Contraceptives (OCs) comprising EE were developed in the early 1960s and EE became a standard component of near all combined forms of contraceptive pills [7]. Despite low hormone doses, in certain cases, OCs may induce serious and even life threatening arterial or venous thromboembolic complications [10]. Since EE was regarded as a bioidentical estrogen, thromboembolic events in OC users were attributed to be characteristic of increased endogenous estrogen levels.

The use of OCs exhibits ambiguous correlations with cancer risk depending on the regulatory features of affected organs [9]. In OC user women, overall breast cancer risk is slightly increased [11 - 13], whilst endometrial and ovarian cancer risks are strongly reduced [14, 15]. These highly controversial correlations between OC use and an increased cancer prevalence at different sites strongly suggest that EE even in low doses is not a pure agonist of ERs, but rather it is an endocrine disruptor inducing alterations in estrogen regulated genes [2].

During the progress of Hormone Replacement Therapy (HRT) for postmenopausal women, both natural estrogens extracted from biological samples and different synthetic hormones; estrogens and progestins were prescribed [4]. Among postmenopausal women, the use of both natural and synthetic estrogens and even their combinations with various synthetic progestins resulted in a chaos of quite controversial clinical experiences. Considering the induction of adverse effects among HRT users; the increased risk for thromboembolic complications and cancers suggests rather a deregulation of genomic mechanisms via synthetic hormone treatment instead of excessive activation of ERs [9]. In a healthy pregnancy, abundant endogenous estrogen supply ensures DNA stability for the abruptly proliferating maternal organs and fetal structures, rather than inducing toxic and tumor promoting impacts [16].

In breast cancer cell lines treated with synthetic estradiol, a paradox of estrogen induced cell growth and apoptosis may be experienced [17]. These observations, together with the controversial findings experienced in HRT user women and HDE treated breast cancer cases, strongly suggested that even endogenous estrogens may have ambiguous tumor promoting and tumor inhibitory activities.

The presented study analyzes all controversial effects of synthetic estrogen use either as HDE treatment for breast cancer or as oral contraceptive pills. Moreover, the risks and benefits of HRT use are reconsidered in the light of applied hormone formulas. All toxic complications of synthetic estrogen use and the ambiguous effects on cancer risk may be explained via understanding the deregulation of ER activation by synthetic estrogen treatment affecting ambiguously both healthy and malignant cells.

2. ENDOGENOUS ESTROGENS UPREGULATE ALL PHYSIOLOGICAL FUNCTIONS OF HEALTHY CELLS, WHILE THEY INDUCE APOPTOTIC DEATH IN TUMOR CELLS

The transcriptional activation of ERs drives the expression of estrogen regulated genes so as to initiate, complete and supervise the replication and recombination of DNA [18]. There is a unique upregulative feedback mechanism between estrogens and ERs. Both high and low estrogen levels induce an increased expression and transcriptional activity of ERs so as to restore or increase cellular ER signaling. In turn, both low and high ER expressions induce powerful estrogen synthesis for the improvement or appropriate augmentation of the crucial ER signaling [19, 20]. High estrogen concentrations increase the expression and activation of ERs, genome stabilizer proteins and aromatase in a circuit upregulating both ER signaling and DNA stabilization. The DNA protective circuit induced by high estrogen concentrations stimulates all physiologic functions of healthy cells, while suppressing the survival possibility of cancer cells in a Janus-faced manner.

In an estrogen deficient milieu, the possibility of unliganded ER activation provides immense reserve capacities for the transient stabilization of genomic machinery [21, 22]. Loss of estrogen endangers the liganded ER activation, while a prompt compensatory upregulation of unliganded ER activation may save the surveillance of the genomic machinery.

Estrogen hormones induce a balanced activation of both estrogen liganded and unliganded (growth factor receptor mediated) transactivation functions of ERs [9]. Estrogen activated ER alpha regulates the expression and activation of growth factors and their membrane associated receptors promoting even the unliganded activation of ERs [23]. Experimental studies revealed a strong interplay between liganded and unliganded transcriptional activations of ERs [24]. Artificial inhibition of either liganded or unliganded ER activation provokes a strong compensatory upregulation on the unaffected domain. In adult men and women, the ligand dependent AF2 activation of ERs enjoys a conspicuous primacy over unliganded AF1 activation. A moderately defective function of AF2 domain may be restored by the activated AF1 domain, while a complete blockade of the superior AF2 domain may not be compensated even in a strongly estrogen rich milieu.

3. MOLECULAR MECHANISM OF ESTROGEN INDUCED SELF REGULATED DEATH IN CANCER CELLS

In tumor cells, estrogen treatment results in a strong upregulation of ER signaling inducing the restoration of genome stabilizer circuit and a concomitant apoptotic death [20].

In tumor cells, estradiol stimulates both liganded and unliganded pathways of ER activation. In ER-positive breast cancer cell lines, estrogen treatment increases the expression and transcriptional activity of ERs as compared with those of untreated controls [25]. Similarly, estradiol administration increases the expression and activity of membrane associated ER-alpha through the phosphatidylinositol 3-kinase (PI 3-K)/Akt system [26]. In breast cancer cells, estrogen treatment increased the expression of growth factor receptors (EGFR and HER2) upregulating the unliganded activation of ERs [27]. In conclusion, an amplified crosstalk between ERs and membrane associated growth factor receptors (GFRs) serves as a means for restoring genomic stability in tumor cells and inducing tumor response [9].

In breast cancer cells, estrogen administration induces an amplification of *ESR1 gene* at 6q25 upregulating ER protein synthesis and a restoration of genome safeguarding processes [28]. Patients exhibiting *ESR1 gene* amplification in their tumors experience a longer disease-free survival as compared with those without it [29].

In tumor cells treated with estradiol, activated ERs mediated the transcriptional regulation and increased expression of lncRNAs, including HOTAIR [30, 31]. Increased HOTAIR expression in the tumors of breast cancer cases was associated with lower risks of relapse and mortality than those showing low HOTAIR expression in their tumors [32]. These findings suggest that estradiol induced increased expression of HOTAIR is associated with epigenetic changes in both *ESR1* and BRCA1 genes, promoting ER-alpha upregulation, DNA stabilization and tumor regression [19].

In breast cancer cells, estrogen activated ERs are capable of increasing aromatase expression and estrogen synthesis, which are essential for the increased liganded activation of ERs. Estradiol treatment elevated aromatase activity in a dose-dependent manner when ER-negative tumor cells were transfected with exogenous ER alpha [33]. In breast cancer cells, estradiol may increase the expression of aromatase enzyme by an unliganded activation of ER-alpha and upregulates aromatase activity as well by means of an enhanced tyrosine phosphorylation of the enzyme [34].

High aromatase activity and increased *in situ* estrogen concentrations were found at the invasive front of cancers, where interplay between the tumor and adjacent tissues may define the expansion or regression of cancer [35]. In breast cancer cases, a direct correlation was experienced between the aromatase activity of removed tumor samples and the patient's survival time after surgery [36, 37].

In MCF-7 tumor cells, estrogen treatment induced an increased expression of BRCA1 protein [38]. In turn, BRCA1 protein induces *ESR1*-gene activation upregulating ER-alpha mRNA expression and protein synthesis in breast cancer cell lines [39]. These observations justify that estrogen activated ER alpha and BRCA1 protein work in close partnership in the genome stabilizer circuit promoting a self directed death of tumor cells [19].

4. MOLECULAR MECHANISMS OF THE INHIBITION AND COMPENSATORY UPREGULATION OF ER SIGNALING BY SYNTHETIC ESTROGEN TREATMENT

Diethylstilbestrol (DES) was pharmaceutically developed for medical purposes. Prenatal exposure to DES was associated with various developmental anomalies of the reproductive tract and heart in girls and of the genitourinary tract in boys [40]. DES treatment during pregnancy induced a modest increase in breast cancer risk. In utero exposures to DES have shown an increased risk for breast cancer in women after the age of 40 [41]. Increased breast cancer risk in DES treated patients mistakenly suggested that synthetic estrogens activate the same subcellular pathways that high estradiol level does leading to alterations in all cellular functions, including interactions with DNA [42, 43].

Developmental anomalies and elevated breast cancer risk induced by prenatal exposure to DES may be attributed to a deregulation of ER signaling pathways. DES preferentially disturbs the ancient functions of ERs; the control of development and differentiation in embryonic life [40]. Prenatal exposure to DES provokes alterations in the epigenome of rapidly developing breasts through definite changes in histone methylation. Disturbed expression of estrogen regulated genes may induce tumor development even in puberty and adulthood [44, 45].

In adult female rats an exposure to DES strongly increases the rate of pathological cell proliferation in mammary epithelium. Female, transgenic mice with inactivated AF2 domain of ERs are not responsive to estrogen treatment, while growth factor treatment induced endometrial proliferation in the absence of estrogen via unliganded ER activation [46]. Although DES is a presumed agonist of ERs, DES treatment blocked the uterotrophic response in AF2 inactive transgenic mice via the inactivation of AF1 domain.

Today, DES is regarded as a harmful representative of endocrine disruptor chemicals (EDCs) strongly deteriorating ER signaling and provoking serious epigenomic alterations [47]. Endocrine disruptor compounds including DES show a strong binding to ERs, whereas exhibiting a special toxicological mechanism; higher doses induce linearly more toxic damages as compared with lower doses; however, there are no safety low levels of these chemicals.

5. BOTH SYNTHETIC ESTROGENS AND ANTIESTROGENS DEREGULATE THE BALANCE OF LIGANDED AND UNLIGANDED ACTIVATIONS OF ERS LEADING TO AN ENDOCRINE DISRUPTION

The development of false synthetic estrogens, including EE, may be regarded as a pharmaceutical mistake as they are rather partial antagonists of ER activation instead of being agonists [48]. Low doses of synthetic estrogens exert an inhibitory effect on the ligand independent, ancient AF1 domain, while inducing compensatory activations on the superior, ligand dependent AF2 domain of ERs mimicking an estrogen-like effect. High doses of synthetic estrogens provoke a serious imbalance between the liganded and unliganded activation of ERs resulting in an uncompensated derangement of the genomic machinery.

Estrogen-like effects of OCs comprising low EE doses may strongly reduce the risk of endometrial and ovarian cancers even in women with BRCA gene mutations [49]. In BRCA gene mutation carrier women, OC use provokes a compensatory upregulation of the weak liganded activation of ERs leading to a strong decrease in the risk of female cancers [20]. Conversely, the risk for poorly differentiated breast cancer is increased in genetically challenged OC user women, as the female breast is strongly vulnerable even to a slight imbalance of liganded and unliganded ER activations [9].

High doses of synthetic estrogens induce uncompensated genome wide, chaotic disorders in ER regulated genes leading to serious toxic symptoms and unforeseeable tumor responses [47]. Toxic symptoms of HDE treatment are mistakenly evaluated as obvious concomitants of the excessive activation of many estrogen regulated genes [42]. In reality, in tumor cells treated with HDE, an uncompensated blockade of the AF1 domain of ERs provokes alterations in all cellular mechanism including DNA replication.

The use of antiestrogens as potent anticancer agents is a medical mistake based on an old misbelief suggesting a carcinogenic capacity of high estrogen concentrations [48]. Antiestrogens, either ER blockers or aromatase inhibitors crudely inhibit the superior, liganded activation of ERs strongly endangering the work of genomic machinery [50].

In genetically proficient women, antiestrogen treatment leads to a compensatory upregulation of ER and GFR expressions, as well as aromatase enzyme synthesis transiently upregulating both liganded and unliganded ER activations leading to tumor responses. In contrast, in genetically challenged patients, the chaotic mixture of artificial ER blockade and weak compensatory activation of ERs may lead to toxic symptoms, unforeseeable tumor responses or aggressive tumor growth [19].

In apparently "antiestrogen resistant" tumors, the markedly increased expression of ERs and GFRs may be mistakenly regarded as a switch towards an adaptive survival technique and a key for acquired antiestrogen resistance [27, 51]. In reality, the amplified expression of ERs and GFRs in antiestrogen resistant tumors promotes a strong compensatory increase in both liganded and unliganded activation of ERs even when it is not satisfactory for the restoration of genomic stability and self directed tumor cell death [9].

The pharmaceutical development of endocrine disruptor agents could not achieve appropriate advances in the field of anticancer fight [48]. The use of synthetic estrogens yielded controversial results in cancer therapy attributed to inhibition of unliganded activations of ERs. The anticancer efficacy of antiestrogens proved to be much more ambiguous attributed to an inhibition of the superior liganded activation of ERs. Conversely, natural estrogens are capable of restoring DNA protection even in tumor cells via a harmonized activation of ERs through AF1 and AF2 domains. Natural estrogens may not provoke genomic instability even in sky-high concentrations [48].

6. RECENT PATENTS SUGGEST NEW METHODS FOR IDENTIFYING *ESR1* GENE AMPLIFICATION IN HUMAN CANCER SAMPLES

Activating *ESR1* mutations located in the ligand-binding domain have been identified in samples from untreated, antihormone sensitive and refractory breast cancers. The clinical relevance of *ESR1* gene amplification is strongly disputed with data showing its predictive value for the response as well as for resistance of cancers to endocrine disruptor therapies [28]. In breast cancers treated with endocrine disruptors, *ESR1* gene amplification maybe a compensatory reaction against the blockade of liganded ER activation leading to an abundant expression of ERs. In contrast, in the exhaustive phase of anti-hormone treatment, the amplification of *ESR1* gene may be coupled with a total blockade of available ERs leading to a progressive tumor growth. In conclusion, an amplification of *ESR1* gene in itself is not capable of defining the level of ER signaling and tumor responses to be expected [19].

A recent patent provides *in vitro* methods for assaying the activating mutations of

ESR1 gene affecting different domains of ERs. Breast cancers with acquired activating ESR1 gene mutations exhibited an increased ER expression and maintained sensitivity to antiestrogen therapy [52].

A new invention relates to an *in-vitro* method for the detection of *ESR1 gene* amplification to identify a candidate patient with a proliferative disease of the endometrium or ovary as suitable for hormone treatment. In a further aspect, the invention provides an *in-vitro* method of identifying an individual with a non-cancerous proliferative disease of the endometrium or ovary who is at risk of developing endometrial or ovarian cancer. The invention also provides kits for performing the above methods [53].

In a recent patent, functional alterations of novel mutant *ESR1* gene associated polypeptides (ERs) were analyzed. In one embodiment, the mutant *ESR1* polypeptide has an altered ligand binding and dimerization activity, an altered translocation activity, an altered AF-2 function, and/or impaired ER signaling compared to a wild type *ESR1* polypeptide. In other embodiments, the mutant *ESR1* polypeptide has a constitutively active transcriptional activity compared to a wild type *ESR1* polypeptide [54].

A presented disclosure generally relates to *in vitro* methods and reagents for the diagnosis, prognosis or the monitoring of estrogen receptor alpha (*ESR1* gene) positive breast cancer. The invention differentiates *ESR1* positive breast cancer which is responsive to endocrine therapy and/or *ESR1* positive breast cancer which is refractory to endocrine therapy. The present disclosure also relates to the treatment management of *ESR1* positive breast cancer [55].

Vaccines against an oncogenic isoform of *ESR1* gene and their use were disclosed. Methods of reducing the likelihood of a developing resistance to a cancer therapeutic or preventive agent are provided herein. The vaccine may include a polynucleotide encoding an *ESR1* polypeptide or a truncation, deletion or substitution mutant thereof. Methods of using the vaccine including the polynucleotide encoding the *ESR1* polypeptide to treat a cancer or precancer are also provided [56]. This patent deserves a mild criticism as the oncogenic nature of an *ESR1* isoform is hardly justifiable among laboratory circumstances.

7. INTRODUCTION OF HIGH DOSE SYNTHETIC ESTROGEN THERAPY FOR ADVANCED BREAST CANCER IN THE PAST

From the early 1940's, HDE treatment was regarded as a therapeutic means against advanced breast cancer. In postmenopausal women, this therapy may presumably suppress the hyperactive pituitary gland via a feedback mechanism [57].

From the early 1960's, high doses of DES became the standard of care in cases with advanced breast cancer despite the low response rate of tumors and experienced high toxicity [58]. The ambiguous clinical results of DES therapy strengthened the concept of estrogen paradox mistakenly suggesting that even endogenous estrogens are breast cancer fueling hormones whilst in high doses, they are capable of inducing tumor responses [9].

Characteristic side effects of high dose DES therapy in postmenopausal breast cancer cases were gastrointestinal complaints and complications of cardiotoxicity including congestive heart failure [59]. Further serious side effects of DES treatment was associated with clotting disorders; thrombophlebitis, pulmonary embolism and cardiovascular diseases [60]. Additionally, treatment with DES frequently induced gynecologic symptoms in postmenopausal patients, including uterine bleeding, while in premenopausal patients, anovulation and amenorrhoea were characteristic side effects [57, 59].

EE was developed as bioidentical synthetic estrogen and it also was introduced for the treatment of advanced breast cancer [57]. High doses of EE resulted in low tumor responses ($\leq$ 30%), while the experienced side effects reflected gastrointestinal and cardiovascular toxicity as well as clotting disorders. Abundant toxic side effects of high dose EE treatment were mistakenly attributed to specific damages of genomic machinery associated with high endogenous estrogen concentrations [58].

The experienced adverse effects reveal that both DES and EE are endocrine disruptor agents inducing dysregulation in ER signaling in a dose-dependent manner; the higher the used dose of DES or EE, the stronger is its toxicity. In contrast, natural estrogens exert a balanced genome safeguarding activity even in sky-high doses [9].

Conjugated Equine Estrogens (CEEs) were available containing natural hormones prepared from a mixture of horse urine derived steroids. Nevertheless, CEEs have not been used for the treatment of breast cancer in high doses as they contain many different estrogens with unknown toxicity [7].

8. REVISITED USE OF HIGH DOSE SYNTHETIC ESTROGEN TREATMENT AGAINST ANTIESTROGEN RESISTANT BREAST CANCERS FROM THE 1990'S

In the late 1960's, antiestrogens capable of inhibiting the liganded activation of ERs were pharmaceutically synthesized and experimentally tried as medicaments against breast cancer. In 1971, the clinical use of a non-steroidal selective inhibitor of ERs, tamoxifen was reported for the treatment of advanced breast cancer in postmenopausal women [58]. Although, the tumor response rates induced by tamoxifen and high dose EE treatment were quite similar (33% versus 31%), toxic side effects were less frequent in the group treated with tamoxifen [61]. From that time onwards, tamoxifen was used as the preferred first-line treatment for postmenopausal women with advanced breast cancer and almost completely replaced the use of HDSEs [7].

Aromatase Inhibitors (AIs) also were developed for the therapeutic reduction of liganded estrogen signaling in breast cancer cases via the blockade of estrogen synthesis [62]. AI treatment against breast cancer showed lower toxicity than tamoxifen use since it induced lower rates of thromboembolic complications and endometrial malignancy. Primary or secondary resistance to AI treatment also was observed in women with advanced breast cancer.

ER blockers and aromatase inhibitors block the superior, liganded activation of ERs through AF2 domain, while a compensatory upregulation of unliganded ER activation may induce a transient, inconsistent tumor response in genetically proficient patients [50]. The blockade of the superior AF2 domain is an emergency situation for the genomic machinery inducing compensatory estrogen synthesis, increased ER expression and a consequential tumor response.

After initial successes of antiestrogen treatment, a long term antiestrogen administration led finally to a high proportion of non-responsive or paradoxically growing tumors [63]. Today, a rapid growth of breast cancers treated with antiestrogen is regarded as a presumed "antiestrogen resistance".

Molecular mechanisms of antiestrogen resistance in tumors treated with ER inhibitors were thoroughly studied. Upregulation of ER expression, activating mutations in *ESR1* gene and a crosstalk between abundantly expressed ERs and GFRs were mistakenly regarded as possible survival techniques in antiestrogen resistant breast cancers [64 - 66]. In reality, in tumors treated with an anti-hormone, a compensatory increase in ER and GFR expressions drives the upregulation of genome stabilizer processes; however, it may become ineffective in tumors deregulated by an exhaustive antiestrogen treatment [19, 50].

In the meantime, antiestrogen withdrawal resulted in promising tumor responses in certain antihormone resistant postmenopausal breast cancer cases [67, 68]. Similar "withdrawal response" was an old clinical practice until the 1970's, to describe the paradoxical pharmacology of high dose DES therapy, when it was used for the treatment of metastatic breast cancer [69]. The possibility of tumor responses associated with a withdrawal of either HDE or antiestrogen treatment may justify the beneficial role of a compensatory restoration of ER signaling subsequent to the cessation of treatment with endocrine disruptors.

From the 1990's, the use of synthetic estrogens for the treatment of advanced breast cancer was revisited. HDE treatment showed promising clinical results in patients who were exposed to multiple prior antiestrogen therapies and their tumors became resistant [7].

Although DES and EE in high doses proved to be strongly toxic synthetic estrogens, they were used again for the treatment of postmenopausal breast cancer cases with resistant tumors previously exposed to antihormone therapies. In 2001, Lønning *et al.* reported the efficacy of high dose DES treatment resulting in a 31% objective tumor response rate among breast cancer cases becoming refractory to prior anti-hormone treatment [70]. In 2006, Agrawal *et al.* reported the anticancer capacity of high dose EE treatment among postmenopausal breast cancer cases heavily pretreated with antiestrogens. In about 25% of patients, objective tumor responses were experienced [71].

In 2009, Ellis *et al.* published the data from a randomized study on the comparison of anticancer efficacies of lower and higher doses of synthetic estradiol (SE2) [72]. Among breast cancer cases, use of lower and higher SE2 doses (6mg *versus* 30mg) resulted in quite similarly low objective tumor regression rates (29% versus 28%), while the lower dose of SE2 had a significantly lower rate of serious toxic effects as compared with that of a higher dose. The authors suggested the preference of lower doses in future clinical studies. Experienced toxic effects of SE2 in both high and low doses suggest that it is an endocrine disruptor compound instead of a bioidentical hormone.

In 2014, Chalasani *et al.* published that a short term low dose SE2 treatment of breast cancer patients could reverse antihormone resistance and resensitized tumors to later aromatase inhibitor treatment [73]. In conclusion, synthetic estrogens were considered as a valuable alternative to chemotherapy for the treatment of breast cancer cases refractory to prior antiestrogen treatment in spite of their toxicity and the achievement of low tumor response rates.

In reality, the modest but unquestionable therapeutic results of HDE treatment on antiestrogen resistant tumors may be attributed to the altering pathways of ER inhibition. Synthetic estrogen administration provokes a compensatory upregulation of the previously artificially inhibited AF2 domain via inhibition of the growth factor dependent AF1 domain. Nevertheless, partial inhibition of ER activation through either AF1 or AF2 domain always provokes an unbalanced compensatory upregulation of ER signaling resulting in unforeseeable tumor responses and serious toxic complications [9].

9. ADVERSE EFFECTS OF ETHINYLESTRADIOL USED AS A CONTRACEPTIVE PILL IN MEDICAL PRACTICE

EE was pharmaceutically developed and nominated as a bioidentical estrogen [74]. The drug started being used as an estrogenic component of oral contraceptives (OCs) in the early 1960's. Today, EE may be found in almost all combined forms of OCs, becoming the most widely used synthetic estrogen in medical practice [75].

OCs comprising low doses of EE apparently work well; however, in certain cases OCs may induce serious toxic side effects, such as venous thromboembolism, stroke and cardiovascular diseases [10]. Moreover, a non-significant association between OC use and an increased risk for breast cancer also was reported [76]. OC use is not indicated for women with metabolic syndrome, type-2 diabetes and hypercholesterolemia, with inclination to arterial or venous thrombosis [77] and with an increased risk for breast cancer [78].

Estrogen regulated genes play crucial roles in all steps of cellular glucose uptake, while a defect of estrogen signaling leads to disorders in glucose metabolism and energy expenditure [79]. OC induced deregulation of ER signal transduction pathways lead to an increased risk for disturbed glucose uptake. It was established that no organ may be free from the damaging effects of OCs [77].

Insulin resistance is associated not only with hypertension and dyslipidemia, but also with serious disorders of coagulation and fibrinolysis [80]. Consequently, OC induced insulin resistance maybe in strong correlation with endothelial lesions, thromboembolism and myocardial infarct. In conclusion, the cardiovascular and thromboembolic complications of OC use may be attributed to a dysregulation of ER signaling pathways with concomitantly developing insulin resistance instead of to an excessive estrogen supply [9].

In summary, the experienced adverse effects of OC use may be attributed to the toxic complications of an inadequately compensated ER-inhibition justifying that EE works as an endocrine disruptor even when it is administered in low doses.

10. SLIGHTLY INCREASED OVERALL BREAST CANCER RISK AMONG OC USERS

Certain studies exposed a moderately or slightly increased overall breast cancer risk in OC users [78, 81, 82], while others found the risk among OC users nearly equal, or even somewhat lower as compared with the risk observed among never OC users [83 - 86].

Among OC user young girls, who have begun to use pill as teenagers, a slightly increased overall breast cancer risk (OR: ≤ 1.3) was observed [82, 87]. OC use beginning near menarche may strongly disturb the balanced transactivation functions of ERs in rapidly developing young breasts and may lead to epigenetic DNA damage. Recent use of OCs comprising high dose EE was in correlation with increased risk for breast cancer (OR: 2.7), while using OC types comprising low dose EE showed no risk [85]. Long term OC use (≥ 10 years) was associated with a slightly increased risk of breast cancer (OR: ≤ 1.3) [78, 81, 82]. In contrast, in a study, performed on more than 4000 breast cancer cases, either longer periods of OC use, or OC use with higher synthetic estrogen doses did not increase the relative risk of breast cancer [86].

Women with inherited *BRCA1* or *BRCA2* gene mutation are at increased risk of breast and ovarian tumors attributed to defective liganded activation of ERs [20]. In women with BRCA2 mutation, the use of OCs was associated with a slightly decreased risk of breast cancer (OR: 0.94), while for BRCA1 mutation carriers, ever use of OCs was in correlation with a slightly increased risk (OR = 1.20) [88].

Among OC users, an increased prevalence of ER/PR negative breast cancer risk (IRR: 1.65) was observed [89], while the risk for Triple-Negative Breast Cancers (TNBCs) was strongly elevated (OR: 2.9-4.2) [90, 91]. In conclusion, OC use may provoke a stronger dysregulation of ER activation in certain genetically challenged women leading to a particularly increased risk for poorly differentiated tumors [9].

Recent literary data support that overall breast cancer risk is slightly increased in OC users especially in current users [11 - 13]. Correlations between OC use and a significant increase in poorly differentiated breast cancer risk indicate that the health of female breasts requires a strict equilibrium between the activation of both ER domains attributed to their cyclic proliferative activity. Consequently, certain genetically challenged women are highly vulnerable to OC induced dysregulations of ER activation.

11. DECREASED RISK FOR ENDOMETRIAL AND OVARIAN CANCERS AMONG OC USERS

EE in low doses exhibits beneficial cancer preventive effects in female reproductive organs mimicking the anticancer capacity of increased endogenous estrogen concentrations [16, 92].

In women, medium-to-long-term use of OCs (5 years or longer) results in a strong reduction in the risk of endometrial cancer (OR: 0.44) and ovarian cancer (OR: 0.60) [14, 15, 78]. In case of OC use for more than 10 years, the risk reduction shows parallelism with the duration of use, achieving even an 80% decrease in risk for both ovarian and endometrial cancers [93].

In young women with anovulatory disorders, OC use may improve insulin resistance and sex hormone imbalances providing a strong protection against the increased risks for endometrial and ovarian cancers [87, 94]. Among these anovulatory women, OC with a low concentration of EE may induce a strong compensatory upregulation of liganded ER activation resulting in a beneficial, estrogen-like effect on glucose uptake and improving genomic machinery.

Use of OCs strongly reduced the risk of ovarian cancer in women with both BRCA1 (OR: 0.56) and BRCA2 mutations (OR: 0.39) [95] and each year of long term contraceptive use could farther decrease ovarian cancer risk [96]. OC use was recommended as a chemo-preventive measure against ovarian cancers in young women with BRCA mutations [49].

In women with genetic defects of ER signaling, the chemo-protective effect of OC use against endometrial and ovarian cancers may be attributed to the fact that in adult women, the health of endometrium and ovaries may be principally dependent on the liganded activation of ERs. In OC users, low doses of EE induce inhibition of the ancient AF1 domain, while stimulating a compensatory activation of the superior AF2 domain of ERs [9].

12. DECREASED RISK OF COLORECTAL CANCER AMONG OC USERS

Recent studies have reported that OC use strongly decreases the risk of colorectal cancer [97, 98]. The summarized Relative Risk (RR) of colorectal cancer forever versus never OC use was 0.82 gained from 11 case-control studies, 0.81 from seven cohort studies, and 0.81 from all studies combined [97]. A meta-analysis of epidemiological studies was carried out to summarize the relationship between OC use and colorectal cancer risk and to quantify the potential dose-response relation [98]. There was a statistically significant decrease in colorectal cancer risk in association with the duration of OC use.

In conclusion, in the colorectal region, the use of AF1 inhibitor OCs has an estrogen like effect reducing the cancer risk via provoking a compensatory upregulation of AF2 mediated ER activation. These experiences suggest that the health of adult colonic mucosa does not require a strict equilibrium between the AF1 and AF2 mediated ER activations, but rather liganded activation through the AF2 domain has a crucial primacy in the anticancer efficacy.

13. INCREASED CERVICAL CANCER RISK AMONG OC USERS

Among OC users, hormonal factors strongly influence the risk of developing cervical cancer [99]. An IARC multi-centric study established that in Human Papilloma Virus (HPV) positive women, a long-term use of OCs is capable of increasing the risk of cervical carcinoma up to four-fold [100]. In one study, a 10% increased cervical cancer risk for women with less than 5 years of OC use was found, while a much higher, 60% increased risk with 5-9 years of use was established [101]. Moreover, a doubling of the risk was established in women with 10 or more years of OC use. Conversely, after the termination of OC use, the risk of cervical cancer has been found to decrease over time [102].

Estrogen hormone is believed to help the transactivation of viral oncogenes, leading to an increase in viral persistence and gene expression [103]. In contrast, a persistent HPV infection is particularly dangerous among older postmenopausal women suggesting a correlation between estrogen deficiency and high susceptibility to the infection of HPV [104].

There is an unquestionable partnership between OC use and HPV infection for increasing the risk of cervical cancer; however, OC contains a false synthetic estrogen (EE) instead of a natural one. Presumably, HPV infection deregulates the liganded activation of ERs provoking an oncogenic impact in cervical epithelial cells, while OC use concomitantly inhibits the unliganded activation of ERs. Among OC user HPV infected women, the highly increased cancer risk for the cervical epithelium may be attributed to the interplay between EE treatment and HPV infection through a parallel inhibition of liganded and unliganded ER activations. The double inhibition of ER transactivation results in a non repairable dysregulation of the genomic machinery leading to a highly increased risk for malignant transformation.

14. USE OF MISCELLANEOUS NATURAL AND SYNTHETIC HORMONES AS A MENOPAUSAL HORMONE REPLACEMENT THERAPY

Background and history of estrogen and progestin use in women over the past decades as well as guidelines and regimens approved by the US Food and Drug Administration (FDA) were reported in 2005 [4]. From the 1940's, hormone therapy became widely used among postmenopausal women for a variety of reasons, including menopausal symptoms and prevention of chronic illnesses, such as coronary heart disease (CHD) and osteoporosis. Estrogen sales doubled and tripled in the mid-1960's to mid-1970's [4].

In the 1970's, in young women taking oral contraceptives comprising high dose

EE, an excess of clotting disorders, elevated risks of thromboembolism, myocardial infarct and stroke were reported [10]. Considering the clotting risk of synthetic estrogen use, the Coronary Drug Project randomized trial conducted on men with coronary heart disease was stopped although in this study a conjugated equine estrogen was prescribed in high doses (5.0 and 2.5mg/day) [4].

In 1975, an increased endometrial cancer risk was reported in estrogen user women compared with non users [105, 106,]. Among women exposed to exogenous estrogen therapy, the risk of endometrial cancer was 4.5 times higher as compared with control patients [106]. In a great meta-analysis study, unopposed estrogen use was found to be associated with substantially increased endometrial cancer risk, particularly in cases of a long duration of hormone treatment, and this increased risk persisted for several years after its discontinuation [107]. In these studies, hormone use was designated simply as exogenous estrogen treatment without discrimination between natural and synthetic estrogen formulas.

From 1975, there was a dramatic decline of estrogen treatment among postmenopausal women attributed to the increased risks for venous and arterial thromboses and endometrial cancer in estrogen users. In 1978, FDA issued a mandate: by April, all estrogen products, both natural and synthetic should contain warning with messages that estrogen has been proved effective only for menopausal complaints, while carries risks of cancer and thromboembolism [4].

From the early 1980's, estrogen use increased again, attributed to evidence for the opposing effects of progestins on estrogen-induced endometrial alterations [4]. Postmenopausal women on combined estrogen/progestogen treatment exhibited the lowest prevalence of endometrial carcinoma. Moreover, oral contraceptives containing both estrogen and progestogen in each tablet proved to be strongly protective against endometrial cancer [108].

In 1982, a well-retained bone mass was reported among postmenopausal women using a horse urine derived estrogen formula; Premarin (Wyeth Pharmaceuticals, Philadelphia, PA) [4]. In 1984, the National Institutes of Health (NIH) Consensus Conference on Osteoporosis established that estrogens are the most effective means for preventing bone loss [109].

In 1985, highly conflicting reports were published in the same journal regarding the cardiovascular risks and benefits of exogenous estrogen use. The Framingham Heart Study reported an increased risk for stroke, thromboembolism and coronary thrombosis among estrogen users [110]. In contrast, in the same year, the Nurses' Health Study identified a decreased risk for cardiovascular disease among women on exogenous estrogen only therapy [111]. The age-adjusted relative risk of coronary disease in those who had ever used estrogen replacement was 0.5 as compared with the risk in never users. The strong cardioprotective effect found in the Nurses' Health Study may be attributed to a predominance of horse urine derived CEE use.

In 1992, a meta-analysis of observational studies was reported by Grady and associates establishing that in postmenopausal women using exogenous estrogens, an approximately 33% less fatal heart disease was registered as compared with non users [112]. The applied estrogen formulas were miscellaneous. The authors established that considering the higher prevalence of CHD, the benefit of heart protective effect would prevent more deaths than those would be caused by the increased risk of breast and uterine cancers. Hormone therapy was particularly recommended for women who have had a hysterectomy and for those showing a high risk for CHD. In 1992, the American College of Physicians published a position statement proposing that all postmenopausal women should use hormone treatment for the prevention of heart disease and prolong life [113].

In 1995, the Writing Group for the PEPI Trial published favorable effects of estrogen or estrogen/progestin regimens on reducing heart disease risk factors among postmenopausal women [114]. Unopposed CEE proved to be an optimal regimen for the elevation of HDL-cholesterol level, but the high rate of endometrial hyperplasia (no cancer) restricted its use to women without a uterus. In women with a uterus, CEE with cyclic progesterone (MP) treatment has the most favorable effect on HDL-C and induced no excess risk of endometrial hyperplasia. These reports promoted increased use of hormone treatment among postmenopausal women through the 1990's. By 2001, approximately 15 million US women were using estrogen therapy, with or without progestins [4].

In 1998, a new meta-analysis study summarized that unopposed estrogen therapy clearly increases the risk for endometrial hyperplasia and cancer, as well as arterial and venous thromboembolic events. Moreover, a long-term estrogen use probably also increases the risk of breast cancer. It was established that randomized trials could not reassuringly confirm the benefit of estrogen therapy for the prevention of CHD, and it should not be recommended to all postmenopausal women [115]. This meta-analysis summarized the results of different studies comprising women treated with miscellaneous estrogen formulas either alone or combined with progestins.

In 2000, the results of a population based case control study were reported on the effects of HRT on women's risk for developing breast cancer. This study provided evidence that the addition of progestin to estrogen treatment enhances the risk for breast cancer relative to estrogen use alone (RR = 2.07 vs. 1.42) [116]. In the majority of estrogen users, an unopposed conjugated equine estrogen was applied in relatively low doses (0.625mg), while in combined HRT users; MPA was a preferential progestin regimen.

In 2002, the Women's Health Initiative (WHI) study was abruptly stopped after reporting a greater harm than benefit of combined CEE plus MPA treatment (PremarinPro, Pfizer) [117]. The results of the study established damaging effects of combined estrogen/progestin therapy among postmenopausal women, in view of the development of both cardiovascular diseases and breast cancer. This publication resulted in a precipitous decrease in combined estrogen/progestin use and a serious reevaluation of menopausal hormone therapy, as the harms of hormone use seemed to outweigh the benefits [4].

In 2003, the results of Million Women Study in the UK were reported on the effects of specific types of HRT on incident and fatal breast cancer. The use of HRT by women aged 50-64 years in the UK over the past decade has resulted in an increased risk of both incident and fatal breast cancer; the risk was three times greater for users of estrogen-progestin combinations than for unopposed estrogen users [118]. These results suggested that progestin formulas may be much more dangerous for the health of female breasts than estrogens. Later, Sweetland *et al.* reported that the risk for venous thromboembolism was significantly greater for women using oral estrogen-progestin regimen than for those using unopposed oral estrogen therapy (RR = 2.07 vs. 1.42). Formulations containing medroxyprogesterone acetate exhibited especially close correlations with an increased prevalence of venous thromboembolism [119].

In 2004, results of a randomized placebo controlled WHI study on the influence of menopausal HRT on the risks of chronic diseases were reported. 10739 postmenopausal women aged 50 to 79 years with prior hysterectomy were treated with 1 dose and 1 schedule of oral conjugated equine estrogen (Premarin 0.625mg/day). After a median follow up of 5.9 years, the incidence of breast cancer was lower in the estrogen group, as compared with the placebo group (HR: 0.77) [120]. The authors could hardly believe the beneficial effect of unopposed Premarin treatment against breast cancer and suggested further investigations.

In 2011, WHI investigators published the results of an extended, 10.7 years follow-up study continued after 5.9 years of Premarin use [121]. The follow up study included 7645 survivor cases out of the 10739 postmenopausal participants of the previous study. Among postmenopausal women without a uterus followed up for 10.7 years, a previous Premarin use resulted in a reduction in breast cancer incidence. The lower incidence of breast cancer seen among women randomized to Premarin group during the previous study became statistically significant with the extended period of follow-up. The long term benefit of Premarin for women's health may be unique and may not be applied to other (synthetic) estrogen formulas.

In 2010, Ragaz *et al.* at the 33rd Annual CTRC-AACR San Antonio Breast Cancer Symposium reported quite opposite results, based on the reanalyzed and reevaluated data of the WHI hormone replacement therapy trial published in 2002 [122]. Authors found that in subgroups of women, without a strong family history of breast cancer and having no benign breast disease prior to their HRT trial enrollment, breast cancer risk was strongly reduced by PremarinPro treatment (HR:0.68, HR:0.57 resp.) [123]. In conclusion, among selected women with low breast cancer risk, premarin could oppose even the highly toxic progestin (MPA) and exerted its beneficial tumor preventive effect.

CONCLUSION

In the past century, efforts of pharmaceutical industry for synthesizing bioidentical estrogens were not equivocally successful and resulted in great confusion in the whole medical practice.

Exclusively, synthetic hormones (DES and EE) were used as a HDE therapy of breast cancer, whereas for contraception among young fertile women, principally EE was used as an estrogenic compound. Considering the chemical purity and the well controllable dosage of synthetic estrogens, they seemed to be more safe in human practice than using conventional hormones extracted from biological samples.

Despite cautious therapeutic measures, HDE in tumor therapy produced shocking, frequently life threatening toxic complications and the experienced beneficial tumor responses were unforeseeable. EE used in low doses as a component of OCs, induced thromboembolic complications in certain cases and exhibited controversial correlations with either an increased or decreased cancer risk at various sites. All the anomalous effects of synthetic estrogen use are characteristic for endocrine disruptors instead of for an increased physiological activation of ERs. In conclusion, the so-called estrogen paradox experienced in both clinical practice and laboratory experiments may be in close correlation with synthetic estrogen treatment.

In contrast, for menopausal hormone therapy, both synthetic and natural estrogens extracted from biological samples were prescribed. In postmenopausal women, the use of estrogens with different origins and even their combinations with synthetic progestins resulted in quite controversial clinical experiences concerning the risks for arterial and venous thromboembolism and for cancers of breasts and endometrium. Among HRT user women, a separated examination of the effects of natural and synthetic hormones may allow to establish the beneficial effects of unopposed CEE on women's health, whilst the adverse impacts of synthetic estrogens and progestins.

The concept of estrogen paradox was based on clinical studies using DES and EE for the treatment of advanced breast cancer in postmenopausal women. Although high doses of DES and EE provoked similar toxic symptoms and controversial tumor response rates, DES was experimentally identified as being an endocrine disruptor agent, while EE is mistakenly regarded as a bioidentical estrogen even today.

The estrogen paradox experienced on tumor cell lines is associated with synthetic estrogen treatment. It may be explained by the partial ER inhibitor nature of synthetic estrogens and the compensatory upregulation of estrogen signaling. In tumors treated with HDE, an artificially provoked imbalance between the activation of two ER domains may explain high toxicities and the ambiguous responses of tumors.

When a partial ER blockade of synthetic estrogens may be successfully defeated by a compensatory ER activation in tumor cells, an upregulation of estrogen regulated genes improves cellular glucose uptake and a restoration of DNA stability may result in good tumor responses. In contrast, when counteractions against a partial ER-inhibitor treatment prove to be weak in tumor cells, a downregulation of estrogen determined genes disturbs glucose uptake and an associated defect in DNA stability leads to stagnation or even a rapid progression of tumors.

In conclusion, the so-called paradox tumor promotion and inhibition are characteristic only for synthetic estrogen treatment attributed to the deregulation of ER signaling pathways. The presented study reveals that an 80 year period of synthetic hormone prescription may be blamed for the misbelief that ERs exposed to elevated endogenous estrogen concentrations may be deregulated and drive cancer-promoting changes.

CURRENT & FUTURE DEVELOPMENTS

Revelation of the endocrine disruptor nature of synthetic estrogens including DES, EE and SE2 illuminates that all controversial correlations between "estrogens" and breast cancer risk are deriving from the mild or crude deregulation of ER signaling pathways. There is no need of synthetic estrogens either as a high dose therapy against breast cancer or as a component of OC pills in low doses. We should not use poisonous chemicals for the treatment of either healthy or cancer patients, when we have excellent genome stabilizer hormones extracted from biological samples. Naturally extracted estrogens or newly developed truly bioidentical ones are to be introduced into all fields of hormone therapy.

CONSENT FOR PUBLICATION

Not applicable.

CONFLICT OF INTEREST

The author confirms that this chapter content has no conflict of interest.

ACKNOWLEDGEMENTS

The author greatly acknowledges Prof. Atta-ur-Rahman and Dr. Khurshid Zaman, the editors of Bentham Science Publishers, for their invitation to publish a chapter for their Patent Series Book - Topics in Anti-Cancer Research.

REFERENCES

[1]   Beatson GT. On the treatment of inoperable cases of carcinoma of the mamma: Suggestions for a new method of treatment, with illustrative cases. Trans Med Chir Soc Edinb 1896; 15: 153-79.
[PMID: 29584099]

[2]   Suba Z. Causal therapy of breast cancer irrelevant of age, tumor stage and ER-status: Stimulation of estrogen signaling coupled with breast conserving surgery. Recent Pat Anticancer Drug Discov 2016; 11(3): 254-66.
[http://dx.doi.org/10.2174/1574892811666160415160211] [PMID: 27087654]

[3]   Suba Z. Estrogen withdrawal by oophorectomy as a presumed anticancer means is a major medical mistake. J Fam Med Community Health 2016; 3(3): 1081-7.

[4]   Stefanick ML. Estrogens and progestins: Background and history, trends in use, and guidelines and regimens approved by the US Food and Drug Administration. Am J Med 2005; 118(Suppl. 12B): 64-73.
[http://dx.doi.org/10.1016/j.amjmed.2005.09.059] [PMID: 16414329]

[5]   Haddow A, Watkinson JM, Paterson E, Koller PC. Influence of synthetic oestrogens on advanced malignant disease. BMJ 1944; 2(4368): 393-8.
[http://dx.doi.org/10.1136/bmj.2.4368.393] [PMID: 20785660]

[6]   Kautz HD. Androgens and estrogen in the treatment of disseminated mammary carcinoma. JAMA 1960; 172(12): 1271-83.

[7]   Coelingh Bennink HJ, Verhoeven C, Dutman AE, Thijssen J. The use of high-dose estrogens for the treatment of breast cancer. Maturitas 2017; 95: 11-23.
[http://dx.doi.org/10.1016/j.maturitas.2016.10.010] [PMID: 27889048]

[8]   Lindberg BS, Johansson ED, Nilsson BA. Plasma levels of nonconjugated oestrone, oestradiol-17beta and oestriol during uncomplicated pregnancy. Acta Obstet Gynecol Scand Suppl 1974; 32(0): 21-36.
[http://dx.doi.org/10.3109/00016347409156390] [PMID: 4527049]

[9]   Suba Z. Amplified crosstalk between estrogen binding and GFR signaling mediated pathways of ER activation drives responses in tumors treated with endocrine disruptors. Recent Pat Anticancer Drug Discov 2018; 13(4): 428-44.

[http://dx.doi.org/10.2174/157489281366618072012 3732] [PMID: 30027855]

[10]   Lidegaard Ø, Løkkegaard E, Jensen A, Skovlund CW, Keiding N. Thrombotic stroke and myocardial infarction with hormonal contraception. N Engl J Med 2012; 366(24): 2257-66.
[http://dx.doi.org/10.1056/NEJMoa1111840] [PMID: 22693997]

[11]   Hunter DJ, Colditz GA, Hankinson SE, *et al.* Oral contraceptive use and breast cancer: A prospective study of young women. Cancer Epidemiol Biomarkers Prev 2010; 19(10): 2496-502.
[http://dx.doi.org/10.1158/1055-9965.EPI-10-0747] [PMID: 20802021]

[12]   Bhupathiraju SN, Grodstein F, Stampfer MJ, Willett WC, Hu FB, Manson JE. Exogenous hormone use: Oral contraceptives, postmenopausal hormone therapy, and health outcomes in the nurses' health study. Am J Public Health 2016; 106(9): 1631-7.
[http://dx.doi.org/10.2105/AJPH.2016.303349] [PMID: 27459451]

[13]   Mørch LS, Skovlund CW, Hannaford PC, Iversen L, Fielding S, Lidegaard Ø. Contemporary Hormonal Contraception and the Risk of Breast Cancer. N Engl J Med 2017; 377(23): 2228-39.
[http://dx.doi.org/10.1056/NEJMoa1700732] [PMID: 29211679]

[14]   Endometrial cancer and oral contraceptives: An individual participant meta-analysis of 27 276 women with endometrial cancer from 36 epidemiological studies. Lancet Oncol 2015; 16(9): 1061-70.
[http://dx.doi.org/10.1016/S1470-2045(15)00212-0] [PMID: 26254030]

[15]   Beral V, Doll R, Hermon C, Peto R, Reeves G. Ovarian cancer and oral contraceptives: Collaborative reanalysis of data from 45 epidemiological studies including 23,257 women with ovarian cancer and 87,303 controls. Lancet 2008; 371(9609): 303-14.
[http://dx.doi.org/10.1016/S0140-6736(08)60167-1] [PMID: 18294997]

[16]   Suba Z. Triple-negative breast cancer risk in women is defined by the defect of estrogen signaling: Preventive and therapeutic implications. OncoTargets Ther 2014; 7: 147-64.
[http://dx.doi.org/10.2147/OTT.S52600] [PMID: 24482576]

[17]   Maximov PY, Lewis-Wamby JS, Jordan VC. The paradox of oestradiol-induced breast cancer cell growth and apoptosis. Curr Signal Transduc Ther 2009; 4(2): 88-102.
[http://dx.doi.org/10.2174/157436209788167484]

[18]   Maggi A. Liganded and unliganded activation of estrogen receptor and hormone replacement therapies. Biochim Biophys Acta 2011; 1812(8): 1054-60.
[http://dx.doi.org/10.1016/j.bbadis.2011.05.001] [PMID: 21605666]

[19]   Suba Z. Activating mutations of *ESR1*, BRCA1 and CYP19 aromatase genes confer tumor response in breast cancers treated with antiestrogens. Recent Pat Anticancer Drug Discov 2017; 12(2): 136-47.
[http://dx.doi.org/10.2174/1574892812666170227110842] [PMID: 28245776]

[20]   Suba Z. DNA stabilization by the upregulation of estrogen signaling in BRCA gene mutation carriers. Drug Des Devel Ther 2015; 9: 2663-75.
[http://dx.doi.org/10.2147/DDDT.S84437] [PMID: 26028963]

[21]   Curtis SW, Washburn T, Sewall C, *et al.* Physiological coupling of growth factor and steroid receptor signaling pathways: Estrogen receptor knockout mice lack estrogen-like response to epidermal growth factor. Proc Natl Acad Sci USA 1996; 93(22): 12626-30.
[http://dx.doi.org/10.1073/pnas.93.22.12626] [PMID: 8901633]

[22]   Caizzi L, Ferrero G, Cutrupi S, *et al.* Genome-wide activity of unliganded estrogen receptor-α in breast cancer cells. Proc Natl Acad Sci USA 2014; 111(13): 4892-7.
[http://dx.doi.org/10.1073/pnas.1315445111] [PMID: 24639548]

[23]   Hewitt SC, Li Y, Li L, Korach KS. Estrogen-mediated regulation of IgF1 transcription and uterine growth involves direct binding of estrogen receptor alpha to estrogen-responsive elements. J Biol Chem 2010; 285(4): 2676-85.
[http://dx.doi.org/10.1074/jbc.M109.043471] [PMID: 19920132]

[24]   Arao Y, Hamilton KJ, Ray MK, Scott G, Mishina Y, Korach KS. Estrogen receptor α AF-2 mutation

results in antagonist reversal and reveals tissue selective function of estrogen receptor modulators. Proc Natl Acad Sci USA 2011; 108(36): 14986-91.
[http://dx.doi.org/10.1073/pnas.1109180108] [PMID: 21873215]

[25]   Liu S, Ruan X, Schultz S, *et al.* Oestetrol stimulates proliferation and oestrogen receptor expression in breast cancer cell lines: Comparison of four oestrogens. Eur J Contracept Reprod Health Care 2015; 20(1): 29-35.
[http://dx.doi.org/10.3109/13625187.2014.951997] [PMID: 25213195]

[26]   Stoica GE, Franke TF, Moroni M, *et al.* Effect of estradiol on estrogen receptor-alpha gene expression and activity can be modulated by the ErbB2/PI 3-K/Akt pathway. Oncogene 2003; 22(39): 7998-8011.
[http://dx.doi.org/10.1038/sj.onc.1206769] [PMID: 12970748]

[27]   Massarweh S, Osborne CK, Creighton CJ, *et al.* Tamoxifen resistance in breast tumors is driven by growth factor receptor signaling with repression of classic estrogen receptor genomic function. Cancer Res 2008; 68(3): 826-33.
[http://dx.doi.org/10.1158/0008-5472.CAN-07-2707] [PMID: 18245484]

[28]   Holst F, Stahl PR, Ruiz C, *et al.* Estrogen receptor alpha (*ESR1*) gene amplification is frequent in breast cancer. Nat Genet 2007; 39(5): 655-60.
[http://dx.doi.org/10.1038/ng2006] [PMID: 17417639]

[29]   Tomita S, Abdalla MOA, Fujiwara S, *et al.* A cluster of noncoding RNAs activates the *ESR1* locus during breast cancer adaptation. Nat Commun 2015; 6: 6966.
[http://dx.doi.org/10.1038/ncomms7966] [PMID: 25923108]

[30]   Tao S, He H, Chen Q. Estradiol induces HOTAIR levels via GPER-mediated miR-148a inhibition in breast cancer. J Transl Med 2015; 13: 131.

[31]   Zhang J, Zhang P, Wang L, Piao HL, Ma L. Long non-coding RNA HOTAIR in carcinogenesis and metastasis. Acta Biochim Biophys Sin (Shanghai) 2014; 46(1): 1-5.
[http://dx.doi.org/10.1093/abbs/gmt117] [PMID: 24165275]

[32]   Lu L, Zhu G, Zhang C, *et al.* Association of large noncoding RNA HOTAIR expression and its downstream intergenic CpG island methylation with survival in breast cancer. Breast Cancer Res Treat 2012; 136(3): 875-83.
[http://dx.doi.org/10.1007/s10549-012-2314-z] [PMID: 23124417]

[33]   Kinoshita Y, Chen S. Induction of aromatase (CYP19) expression in breast cancer cells through a nongenomic action of estrogen receptor alpha. Cancer Res 2003; 63(13): 3546-55.
[PMID: 12839940]

[34]   Catalano S, Giordano C, Panza S, *et al.* Tamoxifen through GPER upregulates aromatase expression: A novel mechanism sustaining tamoxifen-resistant breast cancer cell growth. Breast Cancer Res Treat 2014; 146(2): 273-85.
[http://dx.doi.org/10.1007/s10549-014-3017-4] [PMID: 24928526]

[35]   Sasano H, Miki Y, Nagasaki S, Suzuki T. *In situ* estrogen production and its regulation in human breast carcinoma: From endocrinology to intracrinology. Pathol Int 2009; 59(11): 777-89.
[http://dx.doi.org/10.1111/j.1440-1827.2009.02444.x] [PMID: 19883428]

[36]   Evans TRJ, Rowlands MG, Silva MC, Law M, Coombes RC. Prognostic significance of aromatase and estrone sulfatase enzymes in human breast cancer. J Steroid Biochem Mol Biol 1993; 44(4-6): 583-7.
[http://dx.doi.org/10.1016/0960-0760(93)90263-V] [PMID: 8476770]

[37]   Bollet MA, Savignoni A, De Koning L, *et al.* Tumor aromatase expression as a prognostic factor for local control in young breast cancer patients after breast-conserving treatment. Breast Cancer Res 2009; 11(4): R54.
[http://dx.doi.org/10.1186/bcr2343] [PMID: 19638208]

[38]   Kininis M, Chen BS, Diehl AG, *et al.* Genomic analyses of transcription factor binding, histone

acetylation, and gene expression reveal mechanistically distinct classes of estrogen-regulated promoters. Mol Cell Biol 2007; 27(14): 5090-104.
[http://dx.doi.org/10.1128/MCB.00083-07] [PMID: 17515612]

[39]   Hosey AM, Gorski JJ, Murray MM, *et al.* Molecular basis for estrogen receptor alpha deficiency in BRCA1-linked breast cancer. J Natl Cancer Inst 2007; 99(22): 1683-94.
[http://dx.doi.org/10.1093/jnci/djm207] [PMID: 18000219]

[40]   Titus-Ernstoff L, Troisi R, Hatch EE, *et al.* Birth defects in the sons and daughters of women who were exposed *in utero* to diethylstilbestrol (DES). Int J Androl 2010; 33(2): 377-84.
[http://dx.doi.org/10.1111/j.1365-2605.2009.01010.x] [PMID: 20002218]

[41]   Hoover RN, Hyer M, Pfeiffer RM, *et al.* Adverse health outcomes in women exposed *in utero* to diethylstilbestrol. N Engl J Med 2011; 365(14): 1304-14.
[http://dx.doi.org/10.1056/NEJMoa1013961] [PMID: 21991952]

[42]   Saeed M, Rogan E, Cavalieri E. Mechanism of metabolic activation and DNA adduct formation by the human carcinogen diethylstilbestrol: The defining link to natural estrogens. Int J Cancer 2009; 124(6): 1276-84.
[http://dx.doi.org/10.1002/ijc.24113] [PMID: 19089919]

[43]   Bhan A, Mandal SS. Estradiol-induced transcriptional regulation of long non-coding RNA, HOTAIR. Methods Mol Biol 2016; 1366: 395-412.
[http://dx.doi.org/10.1007/978-1-4939-3127-9_31] [PMID: 26585152]

[44]   Doherty LF, Bromer JG, Zhou Y, Aldad TS, Taylor HS. *In utero* exposure to diethylstilbestrol (DES) or bisphenol-A (BPA) increases EZH2 expression in the mammary gland: An epigenetic mechanism linking endocrine disruptors to breast cancer. Horm Cancer 2010; 1(3): 146-55.
[http://dx.doi.org/10.1007/s12672-010-0015-9] [PMID: 21761357]

[45]   Bhan A, Hussain I, Ansari KI, Bobzean SAM, Perrotti LI, Mandal SS. Histone methyltransferase EZH2 is transcriptionally induced by estradiol as well as estrogenic endocrine disruptors bisphenol-A and diethylstilbestrol. J Mol Biol 2014; 426(20): 3426-41.
[http://dx.doi.org/10.1016/j.jmb.2014.07.025] [PMID: 25088689]

[46]   Sinkevicius KW, Burdette JE, Woloszyn K, *et al.* An estrogen receptor-alpha knock-in mutation provides evidence of ligand-independent signaling and allows modulation of ligand-induced pathways *in vivo*. Endocrinology 2008; 149(6): 2970-9.
[http://dx.doi.org/10.1210/en.2007-1526] [PMID: 18339713]

[47]   Gray JM, Rasanayagam S, Engel C, Rizzo J. State of the evidence 2017: An update on the connection between breast cancer and the environment. Environ Health 2017; 16(1): 94.
[http://dx.doi.org/10.1186/s12940-017-0287-4] [PMID: 28865460]

[48]   Estrogen therapy may still hold the key to fight specific ER resistant breast cancer. Eurekalert. Public release: 01. 08 2018.www.eurekalert.org

[49]   Cibula D, Zikan M, Dusek L, Majek O. Oral contraceptives and risk of ovarian and breast cancers in BRCA mutation carriers: A meta-analysis. Expert Rev Anticancer Ther 2011; 11(8): 1197-207.
[http://dx.doi.org/10.1586/era.11.38] [PMID: 21916573]

[50]   Suba Z. The pitfall of the transient, inconsistent anticancer capacity of antiestrogens and the mechanism of apparent antiestrogen resistance. Drug Des Devel Ther 2015; 9: 4341-53.
[http://dx.doi.org/10.2147/DDDT.S89536] [PMID: 26273195]

[51]   Santen RJ, Song RX, Masamura S, *et al.* Adaptation to estradiol deprivation causes up-regulation of growth factor pathways and hypersensitivity to estradiol in breast cancer cells. Adv Exp Med Biol 2008; 630: 19-34.
[http://dx.doi.org/10.1007/978-0-387-78818-0_2] [PMID: 18637482]

[52]   Chinnaiyan AM, Robinson D, Wu YM. Systems and methods for determining a treatment course of action. WO2015057635, 2015.

[53] Simon R, Sauter G, Terracciano L, Holst F, Lebeau A, Turzynski A. Detection of *ESR1* amplification in endometrium cancer and ovary cancer. US20100210612A1, 2010.

[54] Cronin MT, Frampton GM, Lipson D, Miller VA, Palmer G, Ross JS, *et al.* Novel estrogen receptor mutations and uses thereof. US20170016073, 2017.

[55] Stone A, Zotenko E, Clark S. Methods for diagnosis, prognosis and monitoring of breast cancer and reagents there for. WO2017008117, 2017.

[56] Lyerly HK, Osada T, Hartman ZC. Vaccines against an oncogenic isoform of *ESR1* and methods using the same. US20170196952, 2017.

[57] Kennedy BJ. Diethylstilbestrol versus testosterone propionate therapy in advanced breast cancer. Surg Gynecol Obstet 1965; 120: 1246-50.
[PMID: 14285946]

[58] Stoll BA. Hypothesis: Breast cancer regression under oestrogen therapy. BMJ 1973; 3(5877): 446-50.
[http://dx.doi.org/10.1136/bmj.3.5877.446] [PMID: 4353621]

[59] Cole MP, Jones CT, Todd ID. A new anti-oestrogenic agent in late breast cancer. An early clinical appraisal of ICI46474. Br J Cancer 1971; 25(2): 270-5.
[http://dx.doi.org/10.1038/bjc.1971.33] [PMID: 5115829]

[60] Gockerman JP, Spremulli EN, Raney M, Logan T. Randomized comparison of tamoxifen versus diethylstilbestrol in estrogen receptor-positive or - unknown metastatic breast cancer: A Southeastern Cancer Study Group trial. Cancer Treat Rep 1986; 70(10): 1199-203.
[PMID: 3530447]

[61] Beex L, Pieters G, Smals A, Koenders A, Benraad T, Kloppenborg P. Tamoxifen versus ethinyl estradiol in the treatment of postmenopausal women with advanced breast cancer. Cancer Treat Rep 1981; 65(3-4): 179-85.
[PMID: 7237448]

[62] Lin NU, Winer EP. Advances in adjuvant endocrine therapy for postmenopausal women. J Clin Oncol 2008; 26(5): 798-805.
[http://dx.doi.org/10.1200/JCO.2007.15.0946] [PMID: 18258989]

[63] Bhattacharya P, Abderrahman B, Jordan VC. Opportunities and challenges of long term anti-estrogenic adjuvant therapy: Treatment forever or intermittently? Expert Rev Anticancer Ther 2017; 17(4): 297-310.
[http://dx.doi.org/10.1080/14737140.2017.1297233] [PMID: 28281842]

[64] Tolhurst RS, Thomas RS, Kyle FJ, *et al.* Transient over-expression of estrogen receptor-α in breast cancer cells promotes cell survival and estrogen-independent growth. Breast Cancer Res Treat 2011; 128(2): 357-68.
[http://dx.doi.org/10.1007/s10549-010-1122-6] [PMID: 20730598]

[65] Alluri PG, Speers C, Chinnaiyan AM. Estrogen receptor mutations and their role in breast cancer progression. Breast Cancer Res 2014; 16(6): 494.
[http://dx.doi.org/10.1186/s13058-014-0494-7] [PMID: 25928204]

[66] Osborne CK, Shou J, Massarweh S, Schiff R. Crosstalk between estrogen receptor and growth factor receptor pathways as a cause for endocrine therapy resistance in breast cancer. Clin Cancer Res 2005; 11(2 Pt 2): 865s-70s.
[PMID: 15701879]

[67] Howell A, Dodwell DJ, Anderson H, Redford J. Response after withdrawal of tamoxifen and progestogens in advanced breast cancer. Ann Oncol 1992; 3(8): 611-7.
[http://dx.doi.org/10.1093/oxfordjournals.annonc.a058286] [PMID: 1450042]

[68] Lemmo W. Anti-estrogen withdrawal effect with raloxifene? A case report. Integr Cancer Ther 2016; 15(3): 245-9.

[http://dx.doi.org/10.1177/1534735416658954] [PMID: 27411856]

[69]   Stoll BA. Palliation by Castration or Hormone Administration. Breast Cancer Management Early and Late London, England. W.: Heinemann Medical Books 1977; pp. 133-46.

[70]   Lønning PE, Taylor PD, Anker G, *et al.* High-dose estrogen treatment in postmenopausal breast cancer patients heavily exposed to endocrine therapy. Breast Cancer Res Treat 2001; 67(2): 111-6.
[http://dx.doi.org/10.1023/A:1010619225209] [PMID: 11519859]

[71]   Agrawal A, Robertson JF, Cheung KL. Efficacy and tolerability of high dose "ethinylestradiol" in post-menopausal advanced breast cancer patients heavily pre-treated with endocrine agents. World J Surg Oncol 2006; 4: 44.
[http://dx.doi.org/10.1186/1477-7819-4-44] [PMID: 16834778]

[72]   Ellis MJ, Gao F, Dehdashti F, *et al.* Lower-dose vs. high-dose oral estradiol therapy of hormone receptor-positive, aromatase inhibitor-resistant advanced breast cancer: A Phase 2 randomized study. JAMA 2009; 302(7): 774-80.
[http://dx.doi.org/10.1001/jama.2009.1204] [PMID: 19690310]

[73]   Chalasani P, Stopeck A, Clarke K, Livingston R. A pilot study of estradiol followed by exemestane for reversing endocrine resistance in postmenopausal women with hormone receptor-positive metastatic breast cancer. Oncologist 2014; 19(11): 1127-8.
[http://dx.doi.org/10.1634/theoncologist.2014-0306] [PMID: 25260365]

[74]   Kuhl H. Pharmacology of estrogens and progestogens: Influence of different routes of administration. Climacteric 2005; 8(Suppl. 1): 3-63.
[http://dx.doi.org/10.1080/13697130500148875] [PMID: 16112947]

[75]   Stanczyk FZ, Archer DF, Bhavnani BR. Ethinyl estradiol and 17β-estradiol in combined oral contraceptives: Pharmacokinetics, pharmacodynamics and risk assessment. Contraception 2013; 87(6): 706-27.
[http://dx.doi.org/10.1016/j.contraception.2012.12.011] [PMID: 23375353]

[76]   Brohet RM, Goldgar DE, Easton DF, *et al.* Oral contraceptives and breast cancer risk in the international BRCA1/2 carrier cohort study: A report from EMBRACE, GENEPSO, GEO-HEBON, and the IBCCS Collaborating Group. J Clin Oncol 2007; 25(25): 3831-6.
[http://dx.doi.org/10.1200/JCO.2007.11.1179] [PMID: 17635951]

[77]   Cortés ME, Alfaro AA. The effects of hormonal contraceptives on glycemic regulation. Linacre Q 2014; 81(3): 209-18.
[http://dx.doi.org/10.1179/2050854914Y.0000000023] [PMID: 25249703]

[78]   Urban M, Banks E, Egger S, *et al.* Injectable and oral contraceptive use and cancers of the breast, cervix, ovary, and endometrium in black South African women: Case-control study. PLoS Med 2012; 9(3): e1001182.
[http://dx.doi.org/10.1371/journal.pmed.1001182] [PMID: 22412354]

[79]   Suba Z. Low estrogen exposure and/or defective estrogen signaling induces disturbances in glucose uptake and energy expenditure. J Diabetes Metab 2013; 4: 272-81.
[http://dx.doi.org/10.4172/2155-6156.1000272]

[80]   Yudkin JS. Abnormalities of coagulation and fibrinolysis in insulin resistance. Evidence for a common antecedent? Diabetes Care 1999; 22(Suppl. 3): C25-30.
[PMID: 10189559]

[81]   White E, Malone KE, Weiss NS, Daling JR. Breast cancer among young U.S. women in relation to oral contraceptive use. J Natl Cancer Inst 1994; 86(7): 505-14.
[http://dx.doi.org/10.1093/jnci/86.7.505] [PMID: 8133534]

[82]   Khoo SK, Chick P. Sex steroid hormones and breast cancer: Is there a link with oral contraceptives and hormone replacement therapy? Med J Aust 1992; 156(2): 124-32.
[http://dx.doi.org/10.5694/j.1326-5377.1992.tb126427.x] [PMID: 1736053]

[83]   Gaffield ME, Culwell KR, Ravi A. Oral contraceptives and family history of breast cancer. Contraception 2009; 80(4): 372-80.
[http://dx.doi.org/10.1016/j.contraception.2009.04.010] [PMID: 19751860]

[84]   Iodice S, Barile M, Rotmensz N, *et al.* Oral contraceptive use and breast or ovarian cancer risk in BRCA1/2 carriers: A meta-analysis. Eur J Cancer 2010; 46(12): 2275-84.
[http://dx.doi.org/10.1016/j.ejca.2010.04.018] [PMID: 20537530]

[85]   Beaber EF, Buist DSM, Barlow WE, Malone KE, Reed SD, Li CI. Recent oral contraceptive use by formulation and breast cancer risk among women 20 to 49 years of age. Cancer Res 2014; 74(15): 4078-89.
[http://dx.doi.org/10.1158/0008-5472.CAN-13-3400] [PMID: 25085875]

[86]   Marchbanks PA, McDonald JA, Wilson HG, *et al.* Oral contraceptives and the risk of breast cancer. N Engl J Med 2002; 346(26): 2025-32.
[http://dx.doi.org/10.1056/NEJMoa013202] [PMID: 12087137]

[87]   Deligeoroglou E, Michailidis E, Creatsas G. Oral contraceptives and reproductive system cancer. Ann N Y Acad Sci 2003; 997: 199-208.
[http://dx.doi.org/10.1196/annals.1290.023] [PMID: 14644827]

[88]   Narod SA, Dubé MP, Klijn J, *et al.* Oral contraceptives and the risk of breast cancer in BRCA1 and BRCA2 mutation carriers. J Natl Cancer Inst 2002; 94(23): 1773-9.
[http://dx.doi.org/10.1093/jnci/94.23.1773] [PMID: 12464649]

[89]   Rosenberg L, Boggs DA, Wise LA, Adams-Campbell LL, Palmer JR. Oral contraceptive use and estrogen/progesterone receptor-negative breast cancer among African American women. Cancer Epidemiol Biomarkers Prev 2010; 19(8): 2073-9.
[http://dx.doi.org/10.1158/1055-9965.EPI-10-0428] [PMID: 20647407]

[90]   Ma H, Wang Y, Sullivan-Halley J, *et al.* Use of four biomarkers to evaluate the risk of breast cancer subtypes in the women's contraceptive and reproductive experiences study. Cancer Res 2010; 70(2): 575-87.
[http://dx.doi.org/10.1158/0008-5472.CAN-09-3460] [PMID: 20068186]

[91]   Dolle JM, Daling JR, White E, *et al.* Risk factors for triple-negative breast cancer in women under the age of 45 years. Cancer Epidemiol Biomarkers Prev 2009; 18(4): 1157-66.
[http://dx.doi.org/10.1158/1055-9965.EPI-08-1005] [PMID: 19336554]

[92]   Suba Z. Circulatory estrogen level protects against breast cancer in obese women. Recent Pat Anticancer Drug Discov 2013; 8(2): 154-67.
[http://dx.doi.org/10.2174/1574892811308020004] [PMID: 23061769]

[93]   Mueck AO, Seeger H, Rabe T. Hormonal contraception and risk of endometrial cancer: A systematic review. Endocr Relat Cancer 2010; 17(4): R263-71.
[http://dx.doi.org/10.1677/ERC-10-0076] [PMID: 20870686]

[94]   ESHRE Capri Workshop Group. Ovarian and endometrial function during hormonal contraception. Hum Reprod 2001; 16(7): 1527-35.
[http://dx.doi.org/10.1093/humrep/16.7.1527] [PMID: 11425842]

[95]   McLaughlin JR, Risch HA, Lubinski J, *et al.* Reproductive risk factors for ovarian cancer in carriers of BRCA1 or BRCA2 mutations: A case-control study. Lancet Oncol 2007; 8(1): 26-34.
[http://dx.doi.org/10.1016/S1470-2045(06)70983-4] [PMID: 17196508]

[96]   Whittemore AS, Balise RR, Pharoah PD, *et al.* Oral contraceptive use and ovarian cancer risk among carriers of BRCA1 or BRCA2 mutations. Br J Cancer 2004; 91(11): 1911-5.
[http://dx.doi.org/10.1038/sj.bjc.6602239] [PMID: 15545966]

[97]   Bosetti C, Bravi F, Negri E, La Vecchia C. Oral contraceptives and colorectal cancer risk: A systematic review and meta-analysis. Hum Reprod Update 2009; 15(5): 489-98.
[http://dx.doi.org/10.1093/humupd/dmp017] [PMID: 19414526]

[98]   Luan NN, Wu L, Gong TT, Wang YL, Lin B, Wu QJ. Nonlinear reduction in risk for colorectal cancer by oral contraceptive use: A meta-analysis of epidemiological studies. Cancer Causes Control 2015; 26(1): 65-78.
[http://dx.doi.org/10.1007/s10552-014-0483-2] [PMID: 25359305]

[99]   Roura E, Travier N, Waterboer T, *et al.* The influence of hormonal factors on the risk of developing cervical cancer and pre-cancer: Results from the EPIC cohort. PLoS One 2016; 11(1): e0147029.
[http://dx.doi.org/10.1371/journal.pone.0147029] [PMID: 26808155]

[100]   Moreno V, Bosch FX, Muñoz N, *et al.* Effect of oral contraceptives on risk of cervical cancer in women with human papillomavirus infection: The IARC multicentric case-control study. Lancet 2002; 359(9312): 1085-92.
[http://dx.doi.org/10.1016/S0140-6736(02)08150-3] [PMID: 11943255]

[101]   Smith JS, Green J, Berrington de Gonzalez A, *et al.* Cervical cancer and use of hormonal contraceptives: A systematic review. Lancet 2003; 361(9364): 1159-67.
[http://dx.doi.org/10.1016/S0140-6736(03)12949-2] [PMID: 12686037]

[102]   Appleby P, Beral V, Berrington de González A, *et al.* Cervical cancer and hormonal contraceptives: Collaborative reanalysis of individual data for 16,573 women with cervical cancer and 35,509 women without cervical cancer from 24 epidemiological studies. Lancet 2007; 370(9599): 1609-21.
[http://dx.doi.org/10.1016/S0140-6736(07)61684-5] [PMID: 17993361]

[103]   Mitrani-Rosenbaum S, Tsvieli R, Tur-Kaspa R. Oestrogen stimulates differential transcription of human papillomavirus type 16 in SiHa cervical carcinoma cells. J Gen Virol 1989; 70(Pt 8): 2227-32.
[http://dx.doi.org/10.1099/0022-1317-70-8-2227] [PMID: 2549190]

[104]   Baker R, Dauner JG, Rodriguez AC, *et al.* Increased plasma levels of adipokines and inflammatory markers in older women with persistent HPV infection. Cytokine 2011; 53(3): 282-5.
[http://dx.doi.org/10.1016/j.cyto.2010.11.014] [PMID: 21167737]

[105]   Ziel HK, Finkle WD. Increased risk of endometrial carcinoma among users of conjugated estrogens. N Engl J Med 1975; 293(23): 1167-70.
[http://dx.doi.org/10.1056/NEJM197512042932303] [PMID: 171569]

[106]   Smith DC, Prentice R, Thompson DJ, Herrmann WL. Association of exogenous estrogen and endometrial carcinoma. N Engl J Med 1975; 293(23): 1164-7.
[http://dx.doi.org/10.1056/NEJM197512042932302] [PMID: 1186789]

[107]   Grady D, Gebretsadik T, Kerlikowske K, Ernster V, Petitti D. Hormone replacement therapy and endometrial cancer risk: A meta-analysis. Obstet Gynecol 1995; 85(2): 304-13.
[http://dx.doi.org/10.1016/0029-7844(94)00383-O] [PMID: 7824251]

[108]   Gambrell RD Jr, Bagnell CA, Greenblatt RB. Role of estrogens and progesterone in the etiology and prevention of endometrial cancer: Review. Am J Obstet Gynecol 1983; 146(6): 696-707.
[http://dx.doi.org/10.1016/0002-9378(83)91014-1] [PMID: 6307050]

[109]   Osteoporosis. NIH Consens Dev Conf Consens Statement Online 1984 Apr 2-4 [cited year month day]. 5(3): 1-6.

[110]   Wilson PWF, Garrison RJ, Castelli WP. Postmenopausal estrogen use, cigarette smoking, and cardiovascular morbidity in women over 50. The Framingham Study. N Engl J Med 1985; 313(17): 1038-43.
[http://dx.doi.org/10.1056/NEJM198510243131702] [PMID: 2995808]

[111]   Stampfer MJ, Willett WC, Colditz GA, Rosner B, Speizer FE, Hennekens CH. A prospective study of postmenopausal estrogen therapy and coronary heart disease. N Engl J Med 1985; 313(17): 1044-9.
[http://dx.doi.org/10.1056/NEJM198510243131703] [PMID: 4047106]

[112]   Grady D, Rubin SM, Petitti DB, *et al.* Hormone therapy to prevent disease and prolong life in postmenopausal women. Ann Intern Med 1992; 117(12): 1016-37.
[http://dx.doi.org/10.7326/0003-4819-117-12-1016] [PMID: 1443971]

[113] Guidelines for counseling postmenopausal women about preventive hormone therapy. Ann Intern Med 1992; 117(12): 1038-41.
[http://dx.doi.org/10.7326/0003-4819-117-12-1038] [PMID: 1443972]

[114] Miller VT, LaRosa J, Barnabei V, *et al.* Effects of estrogen or estrogen/progestin regimens on heart disease risk factors in postmenopausal women. The Postmenopausal Estrogen/Progestin Interventions (PEPI) Trial. JAMA 1995; 273(3): 199-208.
[http://dx.doi.org/10.1001/jama.1995.03520270033028] [PMID: 7807658]

[115] Barrett-Connor E, Grady D. Hormone replacement therapy, heart disease, and other considerations. Annu Rev Public Health 1998; 19: 55-72.
[http://dx.doi.org/10.1146/annurev.publhealth.19.1.55] [PMID: 9611612]

[116] Ross RK, Paganini-Hill A, Wan PC, Pike MC. Effect of hormone replacement therapy on breast cancer risk: Estrogen versus estrogen plus progestin. J Natl Cancer Inst 2000; 92(4): 328-32.
[http://dx.doi.org/10.1093/jnci/92.4.328] [PMID: 10675382]

[117] Rossouw JE, Anderson GL, Prentice RL, *et al.* Risks and benefits of estrogen plus progestin in healthy postmenopausal women: Principal results from the Women's Health Initiative randomized controlled trial. JAMA 2002; 288(3): 321-33.
[http://dx.doi.org/10.1001/jama.288.3.321] [PMID: 12117397]

[118] Beral V. Breast cancer and hormone-replacement therapy in the Million Women Study. Lancet 2003; 362(9382): 419-27.
[http://dx.doi.org/10.1016/S0140-6736(03)14065-2] [PMID: 12927427]

[119] Sweetland S, Beral V, Balkwill A, *et al.* Venous thromboembolism risk in relation to use of different types of postmenopausal hormone therapy in a large prospective study. J Thromb Haemost 2012; 10(11): 2277-86.
[http://dx.doi.org/10.1111/j.1538-7836.2012.04919.x] [PMID: 22963114]

[120] Anderson GL, Limacher M, Assaf AR, *et al.* Effects of conjugated equine estrogen in postmenopausal women with hysterectomy: The Women's Health Initiative randomized controlled trial. JAMA 2004; 291(14): 1701-12.
[http://dx.doi.org/10.1001/jama.291.14.1701] [PMID: 15082697]

[121] LaCroix AZ, Chlebowski RT, Manson JE, *et al.* Health outcomes after stopping conjugated equine estrogens among postmenopausal women with prior hysterectomy: A randomized controlled trial. JAMA 2011; 305(13): 1305-14.
[http://dx.doi.org/10.1001/jama.2011.382] [PMID: 21467283]

[122] Ragaz J, Wilson K, Frohlich J, Muraca G, Budlovsky J. Dual estrogen effects on breast cancer: Endogenous estrogen stimulates, exogenous estrogen protects. Further investigation of estrogen chemoprevention is warranted. Cancer Res 2010; 70(24): 441s.

[123] Ragaz J, Shakeraneh S. Estrogen prevention of breast cancer: A critical review. Estrogen Prevention for Breast Cancer. Hauppauge, NY: Nova Science Publishers Inc. 2013; pp. 93-104.

CHAPTER 3

Recent Progress of Phenazines as Anticancer Agents

Hidayat Hussain[1,*], Najeeb Ur Rehman[2], Ghulam Abbas[3], Khanzadi F. Khattak[4], Amjad Khan[5] and Ivan R. Green[6]

[1] Department of Bioorganic Chemistry, Leibniz Institute of Plant Biochemistry, Weinberg 3, Halle (Salle) D-06120, Germany

[2] Natural and Medical Sciences Research Center, University of Nizwa, PC 616, Nizwa, Oman

[3] Department of Biological Sciences and Chemistry, University of Nizwa, Birkat Al-Mauz, P.O. Box 33, Nizwa 616, Oman

[4] Department of Chemistry, Women University, Swabi, Swabi 23430, Pakistan

[5] Boyle & Hooke Oxford, Hampden House, Oxford, Oxfordshire, OX44 7RW, UK

[6] Department of Chemistry and Polymer Science, University of Stellenbosch, Private Bag X1, Matieland, Stellenbosch 7600, South Africa

Abstract: Phenazines are nitrogen-containing heterocycles which possess a wide range of biological activities and in particular, cytotoxic effects. Moreover, various phenazines have been prepared having alkyl, amide, carboxylic acid, aldehyde, and pyrano groups. These synthetic phenazines possess significant anticancer effects towards various cancers. On the other hand, only a few natural phenazines have been reported with anticancer effects. This chapter presents a comprehensive overview of the most recent patents related to the phenazines as anticancer agents.

Keywords: Anticancer agent, *in vitro*, *in vivo*, natural phenazines, phenazine, synthetic phenazines.

1. INTRODUCTION

Phenazines are a large class of natural products isolated from various Gram-positive and Gram-negative bacteria, marine organisms and soil [1, 2]. Furthermore, the core skeleton of phenazines is a pyrazine ring which is a nitrogen-containing heterocyclic metabolite [1 - 5]. In the mid-19th century, it was discovered that phenazines are colored compounds [6] and in 1859, Fordos reported the extraction of a blue pigment "pyocyanine" [7, 8]. Since 1859, over

---

* **Corresponding author Hidayat Hussain:** Department of Bioorganic Chemistry, Leibniz Institute of Plant Biochemistry, Weinberg 3, Halle (Salle) D-06120, Germany; Tel: +49-15226728166; E-mail: hussainchem3@gmail.com

Atta-ur-Rahman and Khurshid Zaman (Eds.)

180 natural phenazines (isolated from various natural sources) and over 6000 synthetic phenazines have been reported [1 - 5]. Initially, phenazines were reported from only *Pseudomonas, Streptomyces*, marine habitats and soil [9]. Various phenazines were isolated from *Pseudomonas* strains, mostly as simple carboxyl- and hydroxyl-substituted compounds with some being C_2-symmetric [10 - 20].

Large numbers of phenazines were reported from *Streptomyces* including simple phenazines (carboxyl- and hydroxyl-substituted compounds) [21 - 26] and very complex phenazines (include thioethers, aldehydes, esters and amides) [27 - 37]. In addition, various terpenoidal phenazines having isoprenylated C- or N-side chains were also reported from *Streptomyces* [38 - 46]. Saphenic acid, which is a chiral 6-(1'-hydroxyethyl)phenazine-1-carboxylic acid and various saphenic acid analogs have been reported from *Streptomyces* [47 - 54]. Very few phenazine glycosides have also been reported from *Streptomyces* and interestingly, have been derived from 6-deoxy-L-glycopyranosides [55 - 57]. There are also other genera that produced phenazines viz., *Methanosarcina mazei* [1], *Pelagiobacter variabilis* [1], *Erwinia herbicola* [1], *Burkholderia phenazinium* [10, 58], *Waksmania aerata* [20], and the *Sorangium* species [1]. This chapter will present a comprehensive overview of the chemical diversity and anticancer activities of natural and synthetic phenazines.

2. ANTICANCER EFFECTS OF PHENAZINES IN NON PATENT LITERATURE

The anticancer effects of natural phenazines have been extensively reviewed by Cimmino *et al.* [3]. Among the simple functionalised phenazines, phenazine PD 116,152 (**1**) (Fig. **1**) isolated from *Streptomyces* sp. possesses cytotoxic effects on colon cells (HCT-8) and mouse L1210 lymphocytic leukemia with IC_{50} ~ 0.5μg/mL [27, 28]. Sendomycin A (**2**) containing the enol amide group demonstrated in vivo anticancer effects in the mouse sarcoma 180 model [6, 59, 60]. Furthermore, the terpenoid phenazine named phenazinomycin (**3**) comprising sesquiterpene moiety, was reported from *Streptomyces* sp. WK-2057 [61]. Interestingly, this compound possesses *in vitro* and *in vivo* antitumor potential towards murine tumours [61, 62]. A monoterpene comprising phenazine named lavanducyanin (**4**), isolated from *Streptomyces* sp. showed cytotoxic effects towards two leukemia cells viz., P388 (IC_{50} = 0.09μg/mL) and L1210 (IC_{50} = 0.1μg/mL) [44]. On the other hand, a saphenic acid derived phenazine DC-86-M (**5**) was reported from *S. Luteogriseus,* and the *in vivo* anticancer activity of this compound showed a 64% (p < 0.05) reduction in murine sarcoma 180 growth [49].

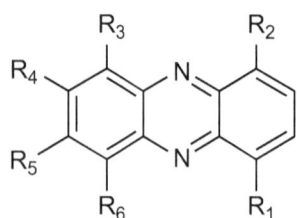

1: R_1: R_3 = R_5 = OH, R_2 = CO_2Me,
R_4 = Me, R_6 = CHO
5: R_1= R_3 = R_4 = R_5 = H, R_2 = CO_2H,
R_6 = $CH(Me)OCOCH_2OH$
6: R_1= R_3 = R_4 = R_5 = H, R_2 = CO_2H,
R_6 = $CH(Me)OCOCH(OMe)CH_2OH$
7: R_1= R_3 = R_4 = R_5 = H, R_2 = CO_2H,
R_6 = $CH(Me)OCO$-2-Me-6-OH-C_6H_3
9: R_4 = R_5 = R_6 = H, R_2 = OMe, R_3 = CO_2H,
R_1 = $CH_2OCOCH(NH_2)C(Me)_2OH$

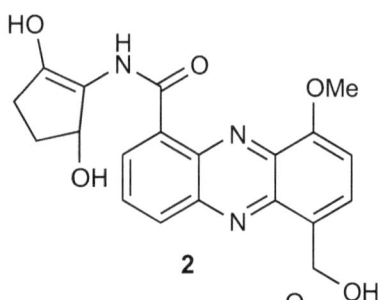

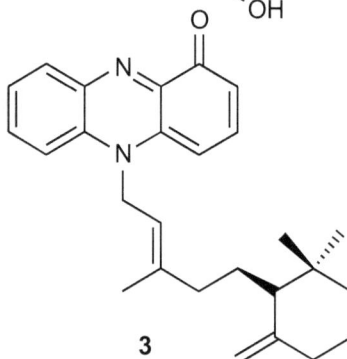

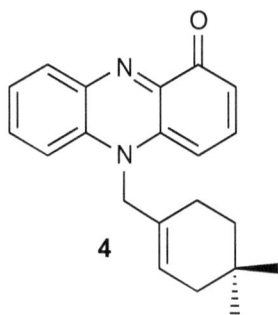

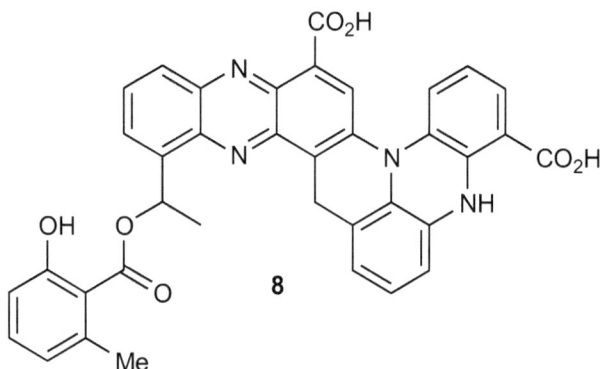

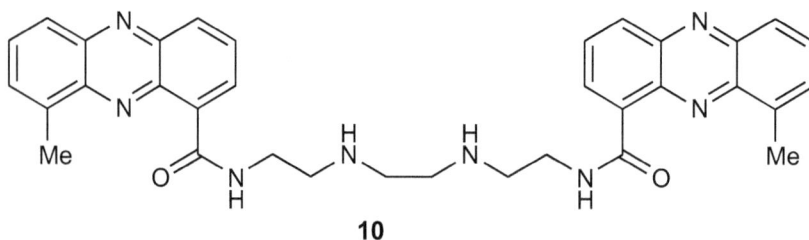

Fig. (1). Cytotoxic effects of phenazines published on non patent literature.

Another phenazine analog DOB-41 (**6**) exhibited *in vivo* anticancer effects in the mouse Sarcoma 180 model but unfortunately was not active in the B16 melanoma and L1210 leukemia models [1, 51]. Another phenazine named (-)-saphenamycin (**7**) reported from *S. canaries* and *S. antibioticus* possesses cytotoxic effects towards the leukemia cells viz., L-5178-Y (IC$_{50}$: 0.15μg/mL) and L1210 and (IC$_{50}$: 0.6μg/mL) [32, 47]. Furthermore, esmeraldine B (**8**) which is a dimeric phenazine, isolated from *S. antibioticus*, possesses good activity towards eukaryotic cells with IC$_{50}$: 0.4μg/mL [63]. Moreover, pelagiomicin A (**9**) reported from the bacterium *Pelagiobacter variabilis* displays cytotoxic effects towards HeLa cells (IC$_{50}$: 0.04μg/mL), BALB3T3 (IC$_{50}$: 0.2μg/mL), and BALB3T3/H-ras (IC$_{50}$: 0.07μg/mL) [64]. Additionally, this phenazine also demonstrated activity against A2780S (IC$_{50}$: 0.2μg/mL), SW620 (IC$_{50}$: 0.5μg/mL), and CCRF-CEM T-cell (IC$_{50}$: 0.7μg/mL) [65].

Various dimeric phenazine-1-carboxamides were prepared and shown to possess significant anticancer effects [66 - 69]. In particular, dimeric phenazine XR5944 (**10**) displays potent *in vitro* and *in vivo* anticancer effects towards a wide range of cancer cells [68, 70 - 76]. In addition, various phenazine-6,11-diones have been prepared and shown to possess significant anticancer effects against various cancer cells [3, 77 - 83]. Furthermore, phenazine-5,10-dioxides, which act as prodrugs for antitumour therapy, have been reported to show promising anticancer effects in various cancer cell [84 - 96].

3. ANTICANCER EFFECTS OF PHENAZINES IN PATENT LITERATURE

3.1. Synthetic Phenazines

In 2017, Lu *et al.* [97] prepared phenazines **11-15** (Fig. **2**) and tested them against various cancer cells interestingly, compound **11** displayed significant effects on colon cancer cells (HCT116: IC$_{50}$: 0.21μM) and also demonstrated activity towards the gastric cancer cell line (MGC-803: IC$_{50}$: 3.4μM), and the lung cancer cells (A549: IC$_{50}$: 6.9μM). On the other hand, phenazines **12** and **15** display promising effects on HCT116 (IC$_{50}$: 1.6 and 2.9μM respectively) with the former compound being effective towards A549 (IC$_{50}$: 2.7μM). Moreover, phenazine **13** and **14** having an amide and carboxylic acid group respectively at C-1, were not effective towards all tested cells. However, compounds **13** and **14** were suitably modified and were then moderately effective towards HCT116 and MGC-803 with IC$_{50}$ < 9μM. In another patent, Gao [98] reported that phenazine **16** displayed significant anticancer effects towards hepatoma cells (HepG2), chronic myelogenous leukemia (K562), HCT116, gastric cancer cell (MGC803), A549 cells, and MCF7 (IC$_{50}$ values were not reported in the published patent).

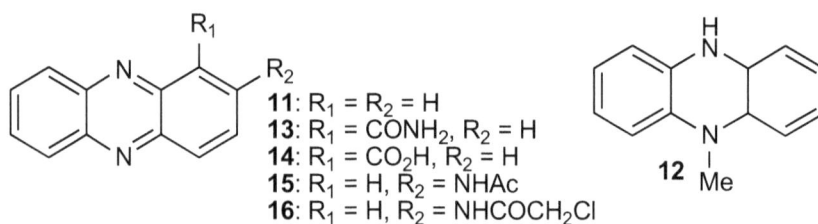

11: R$_1$ = R$_2$ = H
13: R$_1$ = CONH$_2$, R$_2$ = H
14: R$_1$ = CO$_2$H, R$_2$ = H
15: R$_1$ = H, R$_2$ = NHAc
16: R$_1$ = H, R$_2$ = NHCOCH$_2$Cl

12 Me

Fig. (2). Structures of cytotoxic phenazines **11-16**.

Jiang *et al.* [99] prepared a library of pyrano[3,2-α]phenazines **17-36** (Table **1**) and tested these for their anticancer effects. It is interesting to note that compounds **21**, **27**, and **34** possess better activity towards colon (HCT116: **21**: 7.3µM; **27**: 8.0µM; **34**: 8.2µM), breast (MCF-7: **21**: 5.4µM; **27**: 7.3µM; **34**: 10µM), liver (HepG2: **21**: 1.9µM; **27**: 2.1µM; **34**: 2.2µM), and lung (A549: **21**: 9.5µM; **27**: 3.8µM; **34**: 1.5µM) cancer cells. Moreover, all tested compounds demonstrated promising activity towards HepG2 with IC$_{50}$ < 4µM except phenazine **8**. On the other hand, phenazines **18** and **28** showed better effects towards HCT116 with values of IC$_{50}$: 2.5 and 2.6µM, respectively. Moreover, phenazines **22**, **27**, **34-36** possess better activity towards A549 with IC$_{50}$ < 5µM.

Table 1. Structure and Cytotoxic Effects of Pyrano[3,2-α]Phenazine Derivatives 17-36 (IC$_{50}$: µM).

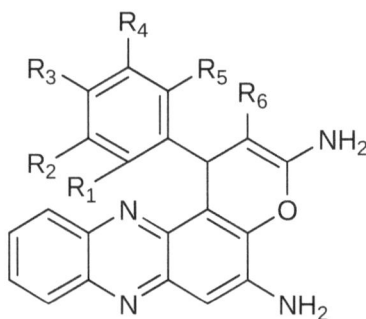

No	R$_1$	R$_2$	R$_3$	R$_4$	R$_5$	R$_6$	HCT116	MCF7	HepG2	A549
17	H	H	H	H	H	CN	19.9	7.1	3.2	20
18	H	H	Et	H	H	CN	2.5	19.1	15.5	23.4
19	H	H	N(Me)$_3$	H	H	CN	12.3	10.9	2.2	8.7
20	F	H	H	H	H	CN	15.1	39.1	3.4	21.4
21	H	H	F	H	H	CN	7.3	5.4	1.9	9.5
22	Cl	H	H	H	H	CN	7.4	25.1	2.4	4.3
23	H	H	Cl	H	H	CN	10.2	11.1	3.2	7.5

(Table 1) contd.....

No	R_1	R_2	R_3	R_4	R_5	R_6	HCT116	MCF7	HepG2	A549
24	NO_2	H	H	H	H	CN	6.4	33.6	1.4	30.2
25	H	OMe	H	H	H	CN	17.6	10.2	2.5	23.1
26	Cl	H	Cl	H	H	CN	10.5	9.3	1.7	11.2
27	H	Cl	Cl	H	H	CN	8.0	7.3	2.1	3.8
28	H	F	OMe	H	H	CN	2.6	> 50	1.8	11.3
29	H	Br	OMe	OMe	H	CN	12.1	25.6	2.2	5.3
30	H	H	$N(Me)_3$	H	H	CO_2Et	14.5	12.2	1.4	7.7
31	NO_2	H	H	H	H	CO_2Et	18.2	18.7	2.4	14.5
32	H	NO_2	H	H	H	CO_2Et	> 50	20.2	2.3	> 50
33	H	H	NO_2	H	H	CO_2Et	16.5	13.2	1.7	18.8
34	H	H	Cl	H	H	CO_2Et	8.2	10	2.2	1.5
35	Br	H	H	H	H	CO_2Et	30.2	28.4	1.4	3.9
36	Cl	Cl	H	H	H	CO_2Et	7.8	> 50	2.1	3.3

Table 2. Structure and Cytotoxic Effects of Phenazine Derivatives 37-44.

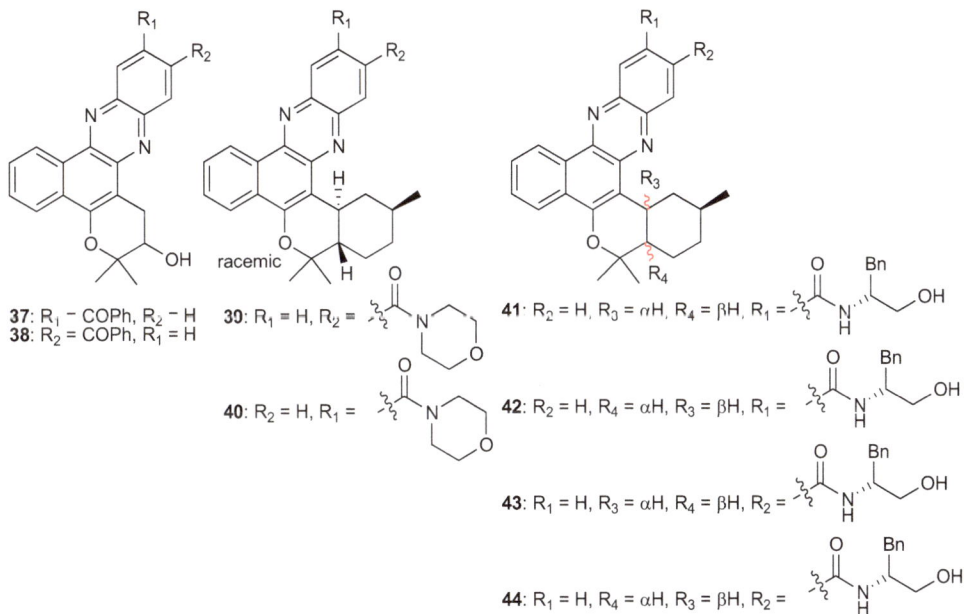

37: R_1 = COPh, R_2 = H
38: R_2 = COPh, R_1 = H

39: R_1 = H, R_2 = [morpholine amide]

40: R_2 = H, R_1 = [morpholine amide]

41: R_2 = H, R_3 = αH, R_4 = βH, R_1 = [amide]

42: R_2 = H, R_4 = αH, R_3 = βH, R_1 = [amide]

43: R_1 = H, R_3 = αH, R_4 = βH, R_2 = [amide]

44: R_1 = H, R_4 = αH, R_3 = βH, R_2 = [amide]

racemic

No	MDA-MB-231	MCF7	PC3	LoVo	siHa	U373
	IC_{50} = μM	Hypoxia 1% O_2				
37+38	1.04	0.46	1.70	1.24	1.20	0.15

(Table 2) contd.....

No	MDA-MB-231	MCF7	PC3	LoVo	siHa	U373
	IC$_{50}$ = μM	Hypoxia 1% O$_2$				
39	1.27	1.45	1.31	1.31	1.13	0.14
40	1.31	1.45	1.41	1.21	1.17	0.61
41+42	11.4	11.0	11.0	9.4	10.5	1.23
43+44	11.0	12.5	11.6	11.4	10.7	1.34
41-44	9.8	6.4	10.5	8.0	11.2	4.1

Feron *et al.* [100] prepared the library of phenazine analogs **37-44** (Table **2**) and evaluated them for their anticancer effects towards breast (MCF-7 and MDA-MB231), cervix (SiHa), prostate (PC-3), glioma (U373), and colorectal (LoVo) cancers. Interesting, a mixture of phenazines **37** and **38** possess remarkable cytotoxic effects towards MCF-7 (IC$_{50}$: 0.46μM), MDA-MB231 (IC$_{50}$: 1.0μM), SiHa (IC$_{50}$: 1.20μM), PC-3 (IC$_{50}$: 1.70μM), U373 (IC$_{50}$: 0.15μM), and LoVo (IC$_{50}$: 1.24μM) cancers. On the other hand compounds **39** and **40** showed similar activity towards MCF-7 (IC$_{50}$: 1.45 vs. 1.45μM), MDA-MB231 (IC$_{50}$: 1.27 vs. 1.31μM), PC-3 (IC$_{50}$: 1.31 vs. 1.41μM), SiHa (IC$_{50}$: 1.13 vs. 1.17μM), U373 (IC$_{50}$: 0.14 vs. 0.61μM), and LoVo (IC$_{50}$: 1.31 vs. 1.21μM), cancers. Moreover, the activity of mixtures **41+42**, **43+44**, and **41-44** were not so impressive towards all tested cancer cells.

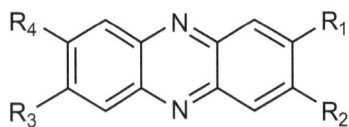

45: R$_1$ = R$_2$ = OC$_{12}$H$_{25}$, R$_3$ = CO$_2$H, R$_4$ = H
46: R$_1$ = R$_2$ = OC$_{12}$H$_{25}$, R$_3$ = R$_4$ = H
47: R$_1$ = R$_2$ = OC$_{12}$H$_{25}$, R$_3$ = CONH(CH$_2$)$_2$NMe$_2$, R$_4$ = H
48: R$_1$ = R$_2$ = OC$_{12}$H$_{25}$, R$_3$ = C(O)OC$_{12}$H$_{25}$, R$_4$ = H
49: R$_1$ = R$_2$ = CH$_3$, R$_3$ = R$_4$ = OH

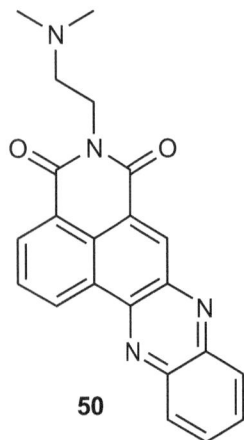

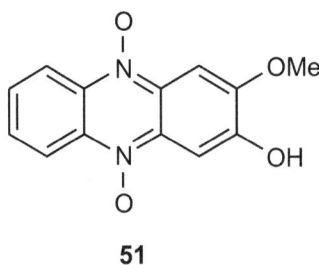

Fig. (3). Structures of cytotoxic phenazines **45-51**.

Camplo *et al.* [101] prepared various phenazines and of these compounds **45-49** (Fig. **3**) proved to display promising activity towards the pancreatic cell (Capan-2), prostate cancer cell (PNT1B, LNCaP, and PC-3), lung cancer cell (A549), colon cancer cell (SW480 and HT290, and breast cancer cells (MCF7 and MDA MB 231). Qian and Yang [102] prepared phenazine **50** and demonstrated that this compound possesses antiproliferative effects on lung cancer, liver cancer, stomach cancer, and leukemia. On the other hand, Takahata *et al.* [103] prepared phenazine **51** which demonstrated significant antitumor effects towards various cancer cells.

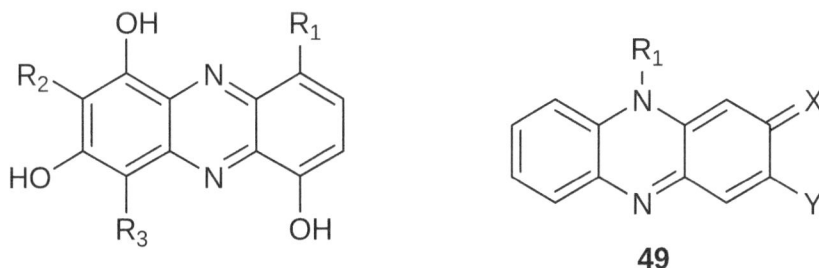

52: R_1 = CO_2H, R_2 = Me, R_3 = CHO
53: R_1 = $CONH(CH_2)_2NEt_2$, R_2 = Me, R_3 = CHO
54: R_1 = $CONH(CH_2)_3NMe_2$, R_2 = Me, R_3 = CHO
55: R_1 = CO_2Me, R_2 = Me, R_3 = $C=N(CH_2)_2NMe_2$
56: R_1 = $CONH(CH_2)_2NMe_2$, R_2 = Me, R_3 = $C=N(CH_2)_2NMe_2$
57: R_1 = $CONH(CH_2)_2NMe_2$, R_2 = H, R_3 = CHO
58: R_1 = $CONH(CH_2)_2NMe_2$, R_2 = Me, R_3 = CHO

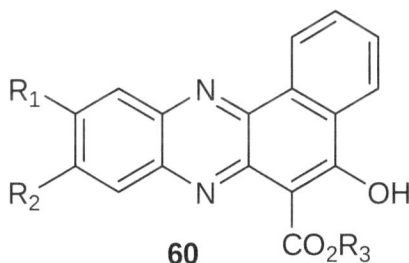

Fig. (4). Structures of cytotoxic phenazines **52-60**.

Bigge *et al.* [104] demonstrated that phenazines **52-58** (Fig. **4**) showed significant cytotoxic activities *in vitro* towards murine leukemia (L1210) cells. Interesting, all compounds possess effects with IC_{50} values ranging from 0.1 to 0.6µg/mL except compound **56** has an which have IC_{50} = 3.4µg/mL. It is noteworthy that compounds **52** and **53** demonstrated activity towards L1210 IC_{50} = 0.17µg/mL. Moreover, these compounds also possess *in vivo* effects towards P388 (murine leukemia) cells. In another patent, Medlen and Anderson [105] prepared various phenazines with formula **59** (R_1 = Ph or substituted phenyl; R_2 = NR_3; H, halogen; R_3 = H, dialkylaminoalkyl and alkyl; X = O, Y = OH] and some phenazines possess promising antiproliferative effects on pharynx caner (FaDu) at $\geq$ 0.25µg/mL. In another patent, Uda *et al.* [106] prepared phenazines with general formula **60** (R^1 = H, OH, halogen, methyl, alkoxy; R^2 = CO_2R^4 (R^4 = H, alkyl, cycloalkyl, benzyl, Ph) and these compounds have been shown to possess antitumor effects towards various cancer cells.

Migita *et al.* [107] prepared phenazine **61** (Fig. **5**) and tested it for anticancer effects. Interestingly, this compound increased the survival time 5.88-fold (at 50mg/kg/day) of mice transplanted with P388 and in the case for 5-FU, the increase for the survival time was 1.76-fold at 25mg/kg/day. In another patent, various 6,11-dihydro-quinoxalino[2,3-g]phthalazine-6,11-dione analogs were prepared and these compounds showed significant cytotoxic effects towards various cancers [108]. Mao *et al.* [109] prepared the platinum complex **62** and this compound has significant activity towards HeLa (IC_{50}: 5.9µM), HepG2 (IC_{50}: 7.1µM), MCF-7 (IC_{50}: 6.3µM), and A549 (IC_{50}: 9.1µM).

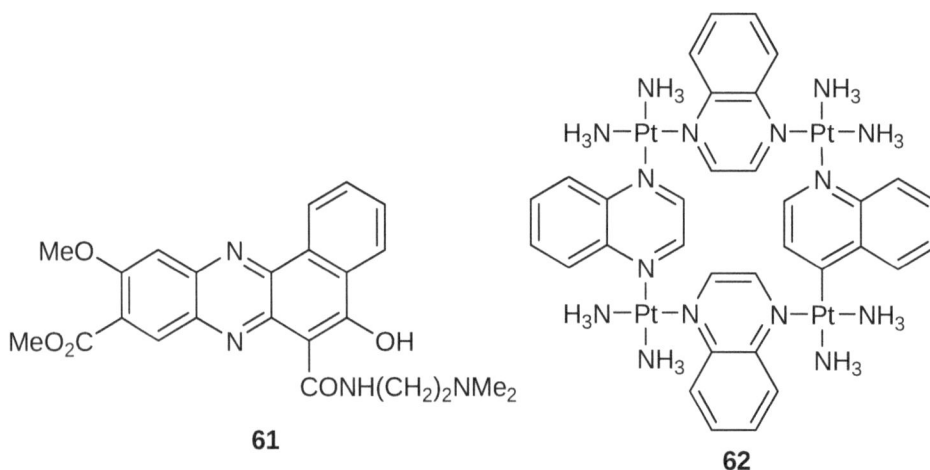

Fig. (5). Structures of cytotoxic phenazines **61** and **62**.

3.2. Phenazine N-Oxides

Døskeland *et al.* [110] prepared various iodinin derivatives **63-71** (Fig. **6**) and tested them against various cancer cell lines. Based on the results, the authors claimed that these compounds may be used to treat acute lymphocytic leukemia, acute myeloid leukemia, chronic lymphocytic leukemia, chronic myeloid leukemia, liver cancer, prostate cancer, breast cancer, bladder cancer, ovarian cancer, pancreatic cancer, adrenal cancer, bile duct cancer, glioblastoma, stomach cancer, bone cancer, neurobastoma, testicular cancer, melanoma, kidney cancer, pituitary cancer, multiple myeloma, brain tumor, colon cancer, esophagus cancer, endometrial cancer, gallbladder cancer, kaposi sarcoma, cervical cancer, thymus cancer, and thyroid cancer.

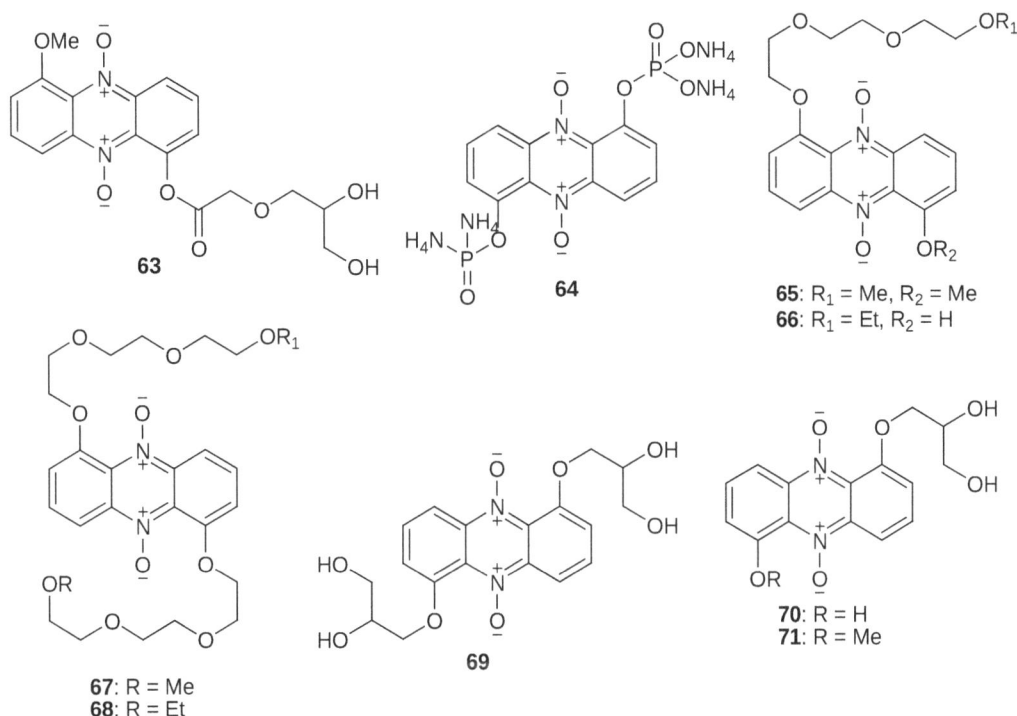

Fig. (6). Strcutures of iodinin derivatives **63-71**.

Rongved *et al.* [111] prepared various iodinin analogs **72-89** and tested them against acute myeloid leukemia cell lines (MOLM-13) and rat cardiomyoblast (H9c2) cells. Initially, iodinin (**72**) was shown to possess anti-neoplastic effects against MOLM-13 (EC$_{50}$ = 0.79 ± 0.10) but was not active towards H9c2 cells. The activity of the prepared compounds is depicted in Table **3**. Interestingly, compound **76**, having an ethylacetate group displayed promising effects towards both MOLM-13 (EC$_{50}$ = 0.38 ± 0.04) and H9c2 (EC$_{50}$ = 1.3 ± 0.2). On the other hand, dimethyl phenazine **81** (*EC$_{50}$* = 0.54) and the dibromo analog **82** (*EC$_{50}$* = 0.70) display significant effects towards *MOLM-13*. However, the latter compound did not display good activity towards *H9c2* (Table **3**).

Table 3. Structures and Anticancer Effects of Iodinin Analogs.

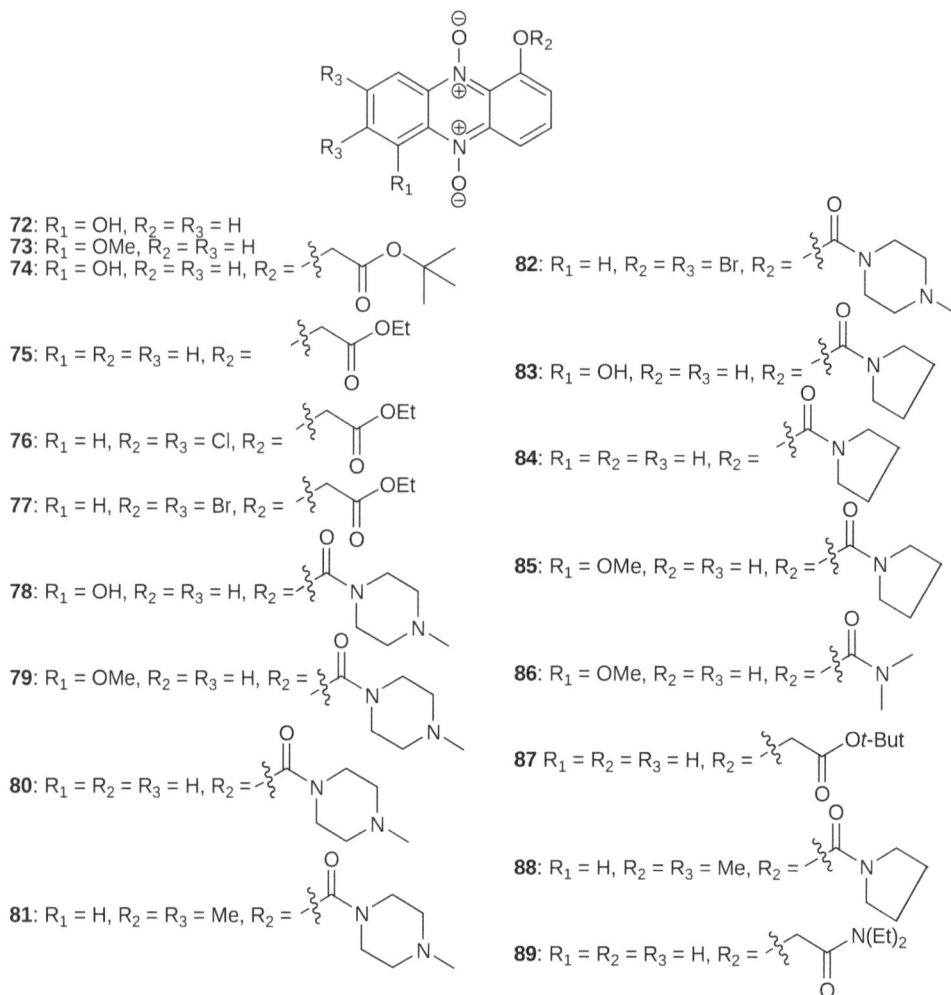

72: R_1 = OH, R_2 = R_3 = H
73: R_1 = OMe, R_2 = R_3 = H
74: R_1 = OH, R_2 = R_3 = H, R_2 =

75: R_1 = R_2 = R_3 = H, R_2 =

76: R_1 = H, R_2 = R_3 = Cl, R_2 =

77: R_1 = H, R_2 = R_3 = Br, R_2 =

78: R_1 = OH, R_2 = R_3 = H, R_2 =

79: R_1 = OMe, R_2 = R_3 = H, R_2 =

80: R_1 = R_2 = R_3 = H, R_2 =

81: R_1 = H, R_2 = R_3 = Me, R_2 =

82: R_1 = H, R_2 = R_3 = Br, R_2 =

83: R_1 = OH, R_2 = R_3 = H, R_2 =

84: R_1 = R_2 = R_3 = H, R_2 =

85: R_1 = OMe, R_2 = R_3 = H, R_2 =

86: R_1 = OMe, R_2 = R_3 = H, R_2 =

87 R_1 = R_2 = R_3 = H, R_2 =

88: R_1 = H, R_2 = R_3 = Me, R_2 =

89: R_1 = R_2 = R_3 = H, R_2 =

No.	MOLM-13 (EC$_{50}$ μM)	H9c2 (EC$_{50}$ μM)	No	MOLM-13 (EC$_{50}$ μM)	H9c2 (EC$_{50}$ μM)
72	0.79 ± 0.10	> 50	73	0.77 ± 0.13	46 ± 4.1
74	0.49 ± 0.12	15 ± 0.9	75	1.29 ± 0.29	20 ± 2.9
76	0.38 ± 0.04	1.3 ± 0.2	77	1.6 ± 0.09	3.3 ± 0.9
78	1.4 ± 0.06	> 50	79	1.4 ± 0.06	26 ± 0.9
80	1.9 ± 0.05	36 ± 11	81	0.54 ± 0.06	9.4 ± 0.55
82	0.70 ± 0.04	> 50	83	0.79 ± 0.09	12 ± 0.79

(Table 3) contd.....

No.	MOLM-13 (EC_{50} µM)	H9c2 (EC_{50} µM)	No	MOLM-13 (EC_{50} µM)	H9c2 (EC_{50} µM)
84	2.1 ± 0.16	16 ± 2.6	85	1.8 ± 0.17	35 ± 3.3
86	1.7 ± 0.09	35 ± 1.8	87	1.9 ± 0.11	20 ± 2.1
88	0.78 ± 0.11	8.7 ± 1.2	89	1.4 ± 0.15	23 ± 0.1

3.3. Natural Phenazines

Li *et al.* [112] isolated phenazine **90** (Fig. **7**) from *Streptomyces* sp. and demonstrated that this compound displayed cytotoxic effects towards the gastric cancer line (BGC-823) and cervix cancer cells (Hela) with IC_{50} = 14.9 and 28.8µg/mL, respectively. In another patent, Ju *et al.* [113] (Table **4**) isolated the two phenazines **91** and **92** from *Streptomyces* sp. and their structures were elucidated by using extensive spectroscopic techniques. Phenazine **91** was active towards glioma (SF-268: IC_{50}: 10.1µM) and MCF-7 (IC_{50}: 16.8µM) while compound **92** displayed cytotoxic effects against MCF-7 (IC_{50}: 21.8µM) and both compounds were inactive against the liver cancer cells (HepG-2) and lung carcinoma (NCI-H460).

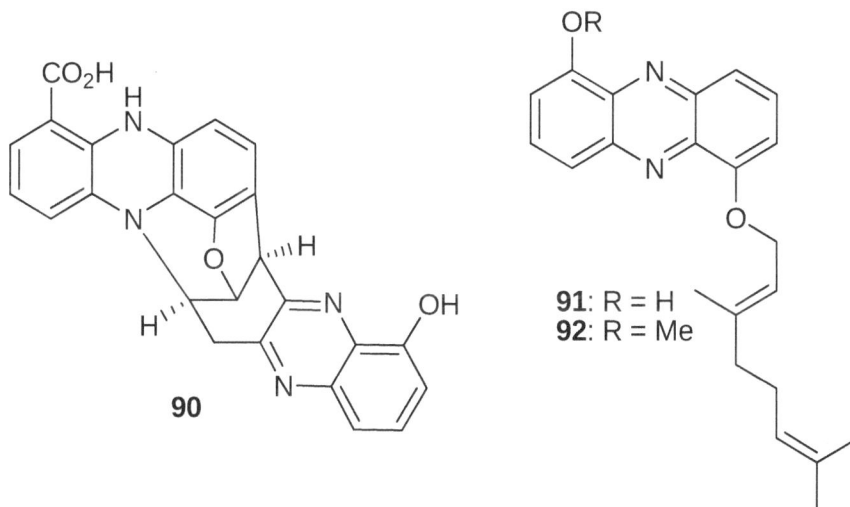

Fig. (7). Structures of natural phenazines **90-92**.

Table 4. Review of Phenazines Patents.

No.	Year	Patent No.	Title	Inventors	Refs.
1	2017	CN106554321	Preparation of phenazine derivatives	Lu, Y., Li, Y.	97

(Table 4) contd.....

No.	Year	Patent No.	Title	Inventors	Refs.
2	2016	CN105418519	Preparation of 2-chloro-*N*-(phenazin-2-yl)acetamide as anticancer agent	Gao, X.	98
3	2016	CN105481869	Preparation of pyrano[3,2-α] phenazine derivatives useful as anticancer agents	Jiang, F., Yan, Y., Lu, Y., Xi, T., Liu, D., Wang, Z., Xing, Y.	99
4	2012	WO2012085222	reparation of novel phenazine derivatives as antiangiogenic and anticancer agents	Feron, O., Riant, O., Kiss, R., Leclercq, J., Chataigne, G., Vandelaer, N., Lamy, C.	100
5	2011	WO2011117830	Derivatives of phenazines useful to treat cancer	Camplo, M., Siri, O., Seillan, C., Iovanna, J., Andrieu, C., Moris, M. A., Rocchi, P.	101
6	2006	CN1880313	Application of heterocyclic dinaphthalimide and its double chained compound for treating tumor cells	Qian, X., Yang, P.	102
7	2006	JP2006241111	Preparation of quinoxalines and phenazines via benzofuroxans	Takahata, T., Sekimura, N., Sumiyoshi, Y.	103
8	1986	EP205339	Antimicrobial and antitumor phenazine carboxaldehydes and derivatives	Bigge, C.F., Elslager, E.F., French, J.C., Graham, B.D., Hokanson, G.C., Mamber, S.W., Smitka, T.A., Tunac, J.B., Wilton, J.H.	104
9	1994	ZA9208419	Phenazine derivatives for treatment of cancer	Medlen, C.E., Anderson, R.	105
10	1988	JP63083073	Preparation of 5-hydroxybenzo[a]phenazine-6-carboxylates as intermediates for antitumor agents	Uda, Y., Kumazawa, Y., Nakagami, Y., Amano, T., Soda, K., Sakakibara, N.	106

(Table 4) contd.....

No.	Year	Patent No.	Title	Inventors	Refs.
11	1986	EP196910	Benzo[a]phenazine derivatives, with antitumor activity, and a process for their preparation	Migita, Y., Eguchi, T., Kumazawa, Y., Nakagami, J., Amano, T., Sota, K., Sakakibara, J.	107
12	2005	KR2005017866	6,11-Dihydroquinoxalino [2,3-g]phthalazine-6,-1-dione derivatives inhibiting cell growth and intermediates and process for preparing them	Kim, J.S., Lee, H.J., Suh, M.E.	108
13	2012	WO2012155559	Organic hybrid tetranuclear Pt complex, preparation method and application in preparing antitumor medicine thereof	Mao, Z., Zheng, X., Tan, C., Huang, H., Ji, L.	109
14	2015	WO2015063516	Compounds	Døskeland, S.O., Rongved, P., Herfindal, L., Borgne, M.L., Viktorsson, E.Ö., Alexander, O., Åstrand, H.	110
15	2018	WO2018109504	Preparation of *N*-oxide heterocycles for use in the treatment of cancer and bacterial diseases	Rongved, P., Aastrand, O.A.H., Viktorsson, E. O., Samuelson, O., Heikal, A.	111
16	2014	CN103993050	Manufacture of novel phenazine antitumor antibiotic with *Streptomyces*	Li, Y., Rong, H., Zhao, L., Xu, L.	112
17	2013	CN103360329	A phenazine compounds and its application in producing anticancer medicines	Ju, J., Song, Y., Huang, H., Zhang, Y.	113

CURRENT & FUTURE DEVELOPMENTS

Phenazines are among some of the most important compounds that have emerged as lead compounds to display a wide range of cytotoxic effects. Furthermore, the phenazine scaffold should be seriously considered as being a "privileged" structure because molecules possessing this scaffold all display interesting biological effects. There are a large number of patents describing synthetic and natural phenazines which support the emergence of these compounds as real alternatives for biologically active compounds. Moreover, an analysis of the patents demonstrated that these compounds are been employed to treat various cancers vis., colon cancer, gastric cancer, lung cancer, hepatoma cancer, leukemia cancer, breast cancer, liver cancer, cervix cancer, prostate cancer, glioma, colorectal cancer, pancreatic cancer, stomach cancer, bladder cancer, ovarian cancer, brain tumor, thyroid carcinoma, and thymus cancer.

It is noteworthy that molecular hybridization has been established as one of the most successful strategies in anticancer drug discovery. Recently, Lu *et al.* [114] reported that pyrano[3,2-a]phenazine hybrid compounds possess significant antitumor effects. Hence, the current authors are of the strong opinion that hybrid compounds of phenazines with other anticancer compounds should be prepared and evaluated since this will not only increase the cytotoxic potentials but could also reduce the side effects associated with anticancer drugs. On the other hand, the current authors further suggest that halogenated phenazines and dimeric phenazines should be prepared and evaluated as we are of the opinion that such molecules would represent phenazines of higher activity.

The authors further noticed that there is a paucity of information about anticancer phenazines used in animal studies and thus suggest that future studies should focus on this aspect more to determine if new active phenazines have been prepared. Although there are a large number of biological applications described for phenazines, the mode of action still needs to be fully investigated. Thus, more information about the toxicity, absorption, and distribution properties needs to be published on phenazines and its analogues to address this question. Unfortunately, *in vivo* studies have been reported for only a few phenazines and additionally SAR studies are not reported in most of the published patents. Therefore, future studies should focus on the *in vivo*, and SAR properties of all active phenazines. Furthermore, in order to discover new anticancer agents to address this debilitating disease, medicinal chemists and biologists should work in collaboration. Finally, the privileged phenazine scaffold has demonstrated itself to be a promising candidate for further chemical manipulation for further libraries of analogues since this will furnish potent therapeutic agents for future clinical studies.

CONSENT FOR PUBLICATION

Not applicable.

CONFLICT OF INTEREST

The author declares no conflict of interest, financial or otherwise.

ACKNOWLEDGEMENTS

The author Hidayat Hussain thanks the Alexander von Humboldt Foundation for its generous support in providing him the opportunity to work in Germany which facilitated the writing of this chapter.

REFERENCES

[1]   Laursen JB, Nielsen J. Phenazine natural products: Biosynthesis, synthetic analogues, and biological activity. Chem Rev 2004; 104(3): 1663-86.
[http://dx.doi.org/10.1021/cr020473j] [PMID: 15008629]

[2]   Guttenberger N, Blankenfeldt W, Breinbauer R. Recent developments in the isolation, biological function, biosynthesis, and synthesis of phenazine natural products. Bioorg Med Chem 2017; 25(22): 6149-66.
[http://dx.doi.org/10.1016/j.bmc.2017.01.002] [PMID: 28094222]

[3]   Cimmino A, Evidente A, Mathieu V, *et al.* Phenazines and cancer. Nat Prod Rep 2012; 29(4): 487-501.
[http://dx.doi.org/10.1039/c2np00079b] [PMID: 22337153]

[4]   Price-Whelan A, Dietrich LE, Newman DK. Rethinking 'secondary' metabolism: Physiological roles for phenazine antibiotics. Nat Chem Biol 2006; 2(2): 71-8.
[http://dx.doi.org/10.1038/nchembio764] [PMID: 16421586]

[5]   Mavrodi DV, Blankenfeldt W, Thomashow LS. Phenazine compounds in fluorescent *Pseudomonas* spp. biosynthesis and regulation. Annu Rev Phytopathol 2006; 44: 417-45.
[http://dx.doi.org/10.1146/annurev.phyto.44.013106.145710] [PMID: 16719720]

[6]   Mavrodi DV, Peever TL, Mavrodi OV, *et al.* Diversity and evolution of the phenazine biosynthesis pathway. Appl Environ Microbiol 2010; 76(3): 866-79.
[http://dx.doi.org/10.1128/AEM.02009-09] [PMID: 20008172]

[7]   Blankenfeldt W, Parsons JF. The structural biology of phenazine biosynthesis. Curr Opin Struct Biol 2014; 29: 26-33.
[http://dx.doi.org/10.1016/j.sbi.2014.08.013] [PMID: 25215885]

[8]   Fordos MJ. Recherches sur la matière colorante des suppurations bleues: pyocyanine. Rec Trav Soc d'Émul Sci Pharm 1859; 3: 30.

[9]   Fordos MJ. Recherches sur la matière colorante des suppurations blue: pyocyanine. C R Hebd Seances Acad Sci 1860; 51: 215-7.

[10]   Turner JM, Messenger AJ. Occurrence, biochemistry and physiology of phenazine pigment production. Adv Microb Physiol 1986; 27: 211-75.
[http://dx.doi.org/10.1016/S0065-2911(08)60306-9] [PMID: 3532716]

[11]   Budzikiewicz H. Secondary metabolites from fluorescent pseudomonads. FEMS Microbiol Rev 1993; 10(3-4): 209-28.
[http://dx.doi.org/10.1111/j.1574-6968.1993.tb05868.x] [PMID: 8318257]

[12]   Leisinger T, Margraff R. Secondary metabolites of the fluorescent pseudomonads. Microbiol Rev 1979; 43(3): 422-42.
[PMID: 120492]

[13]   McDonald M, Mavrodi DV, Thomashow LS, Floss HG. Phenazine biosynthesis in *Pseudomonas fluorescens*: Branchpoint from the primary shikimate biosynthetic pathway and role of phenazine-1,--dicarboxylic acid. J Am Chem Soc 2001; 123(38): 9459-60.
[http://dx.doi.org/10.1021/ja011243+] [PMID: 11562236]

[14]   Hollstein U, McCamey DA. Biosynthesis of phenazines. II. Incorporation of (6-14C)-D-shikimic acid into phenazine-1-carboxylic acid and iodinin. J Org Chem 1973; 38(19): 3415-7.
[http://dx.doi.org/10.1021/jo00959a041] [PMID: 4733458]

[15]   Delaney SM, Mavrodi DV, Bonsall RF, Thomashow LS. *phzO*, a gene for biosynthesis of 2-

hydroxylated phenazine compounds in *Pseudomonas aureofaciens* 30-84. J Bacteriol 2001; 183(1): 318-27.
[http://dx.doi.org/10.1128/JB.183.1.318-327.2001] [PMID: 11114932]

[16]   Handelsman J, Stabb EV. Biocontrol of soilborne plant pathogens. Plant Cell 1996; 8(10): 1855-69.
[http://dx.doi.org/10.1105/tpc.8.10.1855] [PMID: 12239367]

[17]   Sorensen RU, Joseph FJ. *Pseudomonas aeruginosa* as an opportunistic pathogen. In: Campa M, Bendinelli M, Fried-man H, Eds. New York: Plenum Press 1993; p. 43.
[http://dx.doi.org/10.1007/978-1-4615-3036-7_3]

[18]   Parsons JF, Calabrese K, Eisenstein E, Ladner JE. Structure and mechanism of *Pseudomonas aeruginosa* PhzD, an isochorismatase from the phenazine biosynthetic pathway. Biochemistry 2003; 42(19): 5684-93.
[http://dx.doi.org/10.1021/bi027385d] [PMID: 12741825]

[19]   Mavrodi DV, Bonsall RF, Delaney SM, Soule MJ, Phillips G, Thomashow LS. Functional analysis of genes for biosynthesis of pyocyanin and phenazine-1-carboxamide from *Pseudomonas aeruginosa* PAO1. J Bacteriol 2001; 183(21): 6454-65.
[http://dx.doi.org/10.1128/JB.183.21.6454-6465.2001] [PMID: 11591691]

[20]   Gerber NN, Lechevalier MP. Phenazines and phenoxaziones from *Waksmania aerata* sp. nov. and *Pseudomonas iodine.* Biochemistry 1964; 3: 598-602.
[http://dx.doi.org/10.1021/bi00892a022] [PMID: 14188180]

[21]   Chatterjee S, Vijayakumar EKS, Franco CMM, Maurya R, Blumbach J, Ganguli BN. Phencomycin, a new antibiotic from a *Streptomyces* species HIL Y-9031725. J Antibiot 1995; 48(11): 1353-4.
[http://dx.doi.org/10.7164/antibiotics.48.1353] [PMID: 8557581]

[22]   Pusecker K, Laatsch H, Helmke E, Weyland H. Dihydrophencomycin methyl ester, a new phenazine derivative from a marine *Streptomycete.* J Antibiot 1997; 50(6): 479-83.
[http://dx.doi.org/10.7164/antibiotics.50.479] [PMID: 9268003]

[23]   Maul C, Sattler I, Zerlin M, *et al.* Biomolecular-chemical screening: A novel screening approach for the discovery of biologically active secondary metabolites. III. New DNA-binding metabolites. J Antibiot 1999; 52(12): 1124-34.
[http://dx.doi.org/10.7164/antibiotics.52.1124] [PMID: 10695676]

[24]   Tipton CD, Rinehart KL Jr. Lomofungin. I. Degradative studies of a new phenazine antibiotic. J Am Chem Soc 1970; 92(5): 1425-6.
[http://dx.doi.org/10.1021/ja00708a066] [PMID: 5414752]

[25]   Bush K, Henry PR, Souser-Woehleke M, Trejo WH, Slusarchyk DS. Phenacein-an angiotensin-converting enzyme inhibitor produced by a streptomycete. J Antibiot 1984; 37: 1308-12.
[http://dx.doi.org/10.7164/antibiotics.37.1308] [PMID: 6096340]

[26]   Liu WC, Parker WL, Brandt SS, Atwal KS, Ruby EP. Phenacein-an angiotensin-converting enzyme inhibitor produced by a streptomycete. II. Isolation, structure determination and synthesis. J Antibiot 1984; 37(11): 1313-9.
[http://dx.doi.org/10.7164/antibiotics.37.1313] [PMID: 6096341]

[27]   Smitka TA, Bunge RH, Wilton JH, *et al.* PD 116,152, a new phenazine antitumor antibiotic. Structure and antitumor activity. J Antibiot 1986; 39(6): 800-3.
[http://dx.doi.org/10.7164/antibiotics.39.800] [PMID: 3755428]

[28]   Tunac JB, Mamber SW, Graham BD, Dobson WE. PD 116,152, a novel phenazine antitumor antibiotic. Discovery, fermentation, culture characterization and biological activity. J Antibiot 1986; 39(2): 192-7.
[http://dx.doi.org/10.7164/antibiotics.39.192] [PMID: 3754252]

[29]   Gilpin ML, Fulston M, Payne D, Cramp R, Hood I. Isolation and structure determination of two novel phenazines from a *Streptomyces* with inhibitory activity against metallo-enzymes, including metallo--

-lactamase. J Antibiot 1995; 48(10): 1081-5.
[http://dx.doi.org/10.7164/antibiotics.48.1081] [PMID: 7490211]

[30]   Hosoya Y, Adachi H, Nakamura H, *et al.* The structure of diphenazithionin, a novel antioxidant from *Streptomyces griseus* ISP 5236. Tetrahedron Lett 1996; 37: 9227-8.
[http://dx.doi.org/10.1016/S0040-4039(96)02190-9]

[31]   Challand SR, Herbert RB, Holliman FG. A new phenazine synthesis. The synthesis of griseoluteic acid, griseolutein A, and methyl diacetylgriseolutein B. J Chem Soc Chem Commun 1970; 1423-5.
[http://dx.doi.org/10.1039/c29700001423]

[32]   Kitahara M, Nakamura H, Matsuda Y, *et al.* Saphenamycin, a novel antibiotic from a strain of *Streptomyces.* J Antibiot 1982; 35(10): 1412-4.
[http://dx.doi.org/10.7164/antibiotics.35.1412] [PMID: 7174526]

[33]   Nakamura S. Studies on the structure of griseolutein-B, a streptomyces antibiotic. II. Decarboxylation and periodic acid oxidation. Chem Pharm Bull 1958; 6: 543-7.
[http://dx.doi.org/10.1248/cpb.6.543]

[34]   Nakamura S. Studies on structure of Griseolutein B, a streptomyces antibiotic. I. Characterization and degradation. Chem Pharm Bull 1958; 6: 539-43.
[http://dx.doi.org/10.1248/cpb.6.539]

[35]   Nakamura S. Structure of griseolutein B. J Antibiot Ser A 1959; 12: 26-7.

[36]   Nakamura S. Studies on structure of griseolutein-B, a streptomyces antibiotic. III. The complete structure. Chem Pharm Bull 1958; 6: 547-50.
[http://dx.doi.org/10.1248/cpb.6.547]

[37]   Nakano H, Yoshida M, Shirahata K, *et al.* Senacarcin A, a new antitumor antibiotic produced by *Streptomyces endus* subsp. *aureus.* J Antibiot 1982; 35(6): 760-2.
[http://dx.doi.org/10.7164/antibiotics.35.760] [PMID: 7118728]

[38]   Gebhardt K, Schimana J, Krastel P, *et al.* Endophenazines A-D, new phenazine antibiotics from the arthropod associated endosymbiont *Streptomyces anulatus.* I. Taxonomy, fermentation, isolation and biological activities. J Antibiot 2002; 55(9): 794-800.
[http://dx.doi.org/10.7164/antibiotics.55.794] [PMID: 12458768]

[39]   Krastel P, Zeeck A, Gebhardt K, Fiedler HP, Rheinheimer J. Endophenazines A-D, new phenazine antibiotics from the athropod associated endosymbiont *Streptomyces anulatus* II. Structure elucidation. J Antibiot 2002; 55(9): 801-6.
[http://dx.doi.org/10.7164/antibiotics.55.801] [PMID: 12458769]

[40]   Emoto T, Kubosaki N, Yamagiwa Y, Kamikawa T. A new route to phenazines. Tetrahedron Lett 2000; 41: 355-8.
[http://dx.doi.org/10.1016/S0040-4039(99)02061-4]

[41]   Shin-ya K, Furihata K, Hayakawa Y, Seto H, Kato Y, Clardy J. The structure of benthocyanin A. A new free radical scavenger of microbial origin. Tetrahedron Lett 1991; 32: 943-6.
[http://dx.doi.org/10.1016/S0040-4039(00)92126-9]

[42]   Shin-ya K, Furihata K, Teshima Y, Hayakawa Y, Seto H. Benthocyanins B and C, new free radical scavengers from *Streptomyces prunicolor.* J Org Chem 1993; 58: 4170-2.
[http://dx.doi.org/10.1021/jo00067a069]

[43]   Kinoshita Y, Kitahara T. Total synthesis of phenazinomycin and its enantiomer via high-pressure reaction. Tetrahedron Lett 1997; 38: 4993-6.
[http://dx.doi.org/10.1016/S0040-4039(97)01068-X]

[44]   Imai S, Furihata K, Hayakawa Y, Noguchi T, Seto H. Lavanducyanin, a new antitumor substance produced by *Streptomyces* sp. J Antibiot 1989; 42(7): 1196-8.
[http://dx.doi.org/10.7164/antibiotics.42.1196] [PMID: 2753825]

[45]   Nakayama O, Shigematsu N, Katayama A, *et al.* WS-9659 A and B, novel testosterone 5 α-reductase inhibitors isolated from a *Streptomyces.* II. Structural elucidation of WS-9659 A and B. J Antibiot 1989; 42(8): 1230-4.
[http://dx.doi.org/10.7164/antibiotics.42.1230] [PMID: 2759905]

[46]   Nakayama O, Yagi M, Tanaka M, Kiyoto S, Okuhara M, Kohsaka M. WS-9659 A and B, novel testosterone 5 α-reductase inhibitors isolated from a *Streptomyces.* I. Taxonomy, fermentation, isolation, physico-chemical characteristics. J Antibiot 1989; 42(8): 1221-9.
[http://dx.doi.org/10.7164/antibiotics.42.1221] [PMID: 2759904]

[47]   Geiger A, Keller-Schierlein W, Brandl M, Zähner H. Metabolites of microorganisms. 247. Phenazines from *Streptomyces antibioticus,* strain Tü 2706. J Antibiot 1988; 41(11): 1542-51.
[http://dx.doi.org/10.7164/antibiotics.41.1542] [PMID: 3058669]

[48]   Abdelfattah MS, Toume K, Ishibashi M. Isolation and structure elucidation of izuminosides A-C: A rare phenazine glycosides from *Streptomyces* sp. IFM 11260. J Antibiot 2011; 64: 271-5.
[http://dx.doi.org/10.1038/ja.2010.172] [PMID: 21304533]

[49]   Takahashi K, Takahashi I, Morimoto M, Tomita F. DC-86-M, a novel antitumor antibiotic. II. Structure determination and biological activities. J Antibiot 1986; 39(5): 624-8.
[http://dx.doi.org/10.7164/antibiotics.39.624] [PMID: 3733511]

[50]   Asano K, Takahashi K, Tomita F, Kawamoto I. DC-86-M, a novel antitumor antibiotic. I. Taxonomy of producing organism and fermentation. J Antibiot 1986; 39(5): 619-23.
[http://dx.doi.org/10.7164/antibiotics.39.619] [PMID: 3733510]

[51]   Shoji J, Sakazaki R, Nakai H, *et al.* Isolation of a new phenazine antibiotic, DOB-41, from *Pseudomonas* species. J Antibiot 1988; 41(5): 589-94.
[http://dx.doi.org/10.7164/antibiotics.41.589] [PMID: 3384746]

[52]   Kim WG, Ryoo IJ, Yun BS, Shin-ya K, Seto H, Yoo ID. Phenazostatin C, a new diphenazine with neuronal cell protecting activity from *Streptomyces* sp. J Antibiot 1999; 52(8): 758-61.
[http://dx.doi.org/10.7164/antibiotics.52.758] [PMID: 10580390]

[53]   Yun BS, Ryoo IJ, Kim WG, *et al.* Structures of phenazostatins A and B, neuronal cell protecting substances of microbial origin. Tetrahedron Lett 1996; 37: 8529-30.
[http://dx.doi.org/10.1016/0040-4039(96)01983-1]

[54]   Kim WG, Ryoo IJ, Yun BS, Shin-Ya K, Seto H, Yoo ID. New diphenazines with neuronal cell protecting activity, phenazostatins A and B, produced by *Streptomyces* sp. J Antibiot 1997; 50(9): 715-21.
[http://dx.doi.org/10.7164/antibiotics.50.715] [PMID: 9360614]

[55]   Pathirana C, Jensen PR, Dwight R, Fenical W. Rare phenazine L-quinovose esters from a marine actinomycete. J Org Chem 1992; 57: 740-2.
[http://dx.doi.org/10.1021/jo00028a060]

[56]   Kato S, Shindo K, Yamagishi Y, Matsuoka M, Kawai H, Mochizuki J. Phenazoviridin, a novel free radical scavenger from *Streptomyces* sp. Taxonomy, fermentation, isolation, structure elucidation and biological properties. J Antibiot 1993; 46(10): 1485-93.
[http://dx.doi.org/10.7164/antibiotics.46.1485] [PMID: 8244877]

[57]   Kunigami T, Shin-Ya K, Furihata K, Furihata K, Hayakawa Y, Seto H. A novel neuronal cell protecting substance, aestivophoenin C, produced by *Streptomyces purpeofuscus.* J Antibiot 1998; 51(9): 880-2.
[http://dx.doi.org/10.7164/antibiotics.51.880] [PMID: 9820239]

[58]   Garrity GM, Winters M, Searles DB. Taxonomic Outline of the Procaryotic Genera Bergey's Manual of Systematic Bacteriology. 2nd ed., New York: Springer-Verlag 2001.

[59]   Mentel M, Ahuja EG, Mavrodi DV, Breinbauer R, Thomashow LS, Blankenfeldt W. Of two make one: the biosynthesis of phenazines. ChemBioChem 2009; 10(14): 2295-304.

[http://dx.doi.org/10.1002/cbic.200900323] [PMID: 19658148]

[60] Gross H, Loper JE. Genomics of secondary metabolite production by *Pseudomonas* spp. Nat Prod Rep 2009; 26(11): 1408-46.
[http://dx.doi.org/10.1039/b817075b] [PMID: 19844639]

[61] Funayama S, Eda S, Komyhama K, Omura S. Structure of phenazinomycin, a novel antitumor antibiotic. Tetrahedron Lett 1989; 30: 3151-4.
[http://dx.doi.org/10.1016/S0040-4039(00)99188-3]

[62] Omura S, Eda S, Funayama S, Komiyama K, Takahashi Y, Woodruff HB. Studies on a novel antitumor antibiotic, phenazinomycin: taxonomy, fermentation, isolation, and physicochemical and biological characteristics. J Antibiot 1989; 42(7): 1037-42.
[http://dx.doi.org/10.7164/antibiotics.42.1037] [PMID: 2753810]

[63] Keller-Schierlein W, Geiger A, Zahner H, Brandl M. The Esmeraldines A and B, green pigments from *Streptomyces antibioticus*, strain tü 2706. Helv Chim Acta 1988; 71: 2058-70.
[http://dx.doi.org/10.1002/hlca.19880710824]

[64] Imamura N, Nishijima M, Takadera T, Adachi K, Sakai M, Sano H. New anticancer antibiotics pelagiomicins, produced by a new marine bacterium *Pelagiobacter variabilis.* J Antibiot 1997; 50(1): 8-12.
[http://dx.doi.org/10.7164/antibiotics.50.8] [PMID: 9066759]

[65] Singh MP, Menendez AT, Petersen PJ, Ding WD, Maiese WM, Greenstein M. Biological and mechanistic activities of phenazine antibiotics produced by culture LL-14I352. J Antibiot 1997; 50(9): 785-7.
[http://dx.doi.org/10.7164/antibiotics.50.785] [PMID: 9360627]

[66] Garg R, Denny WA, Hansch C. Comparative QSAR studies on substituted bis-(acridines) and bis-(phenazines)-carboxamides: A new class of anticancer agents. Bioorg Med Chem 2000; 8(7): 1835-9.
[http://dx.doi.org/10.1016/S0968-0896(00)00114-0] [PMID: 10976532]

[67] Spicer JA, Gamage SA, Rewcastle GW, *et al.* Bis(phenazine-1-carboxamides): Structure-activity relationships for a new class of dual topoisomerase I/II-directed anticancer drugs. J Med Chem 2000; 43(7): 1350-8.
[http://dx.doi.org/10.1021/jm990423f] [PMID: 10753472]

[68] Gamage SA, Spicer JA, Finlay GJ, *et al.* Dicationic bis(9-methylphenazine-1-carboxamides): relationships between biological activity and linker chain structure for a series of potent topoisomerase targeted anticancer drugs. J Med Chem 2001; 44(9): 1407-15.
[http://dx.doi.org/10.1021/jm0003283] [PMID: 11311063]

[69] Spicer JA, Gamage SA, Finlay GJ, Denny WA. Synthesis and evaluation of unsymmetrical bis(arylcarboxamides) designed as topoisomerase-targeted anticancer drugs. Bioorg Med Chem 2002; 10(1): 19-29.
[http://dx.doi.org/10.1016/S0968-0896(01)00249-8] [PMID: 11738603]

[70] Stewart AJ, Mistry P, Dangerfield W, *et al.* Antitumor activity of XR5944, a novel and potent topoisomerase poison. Anticancer Drugs 2001; 12(4): 359-67.
[http://dx.doi.org/10.1097/00001813-200104000-00009] [PMID: 11335793]

[71] Di Nicolantonio F, Knight LA, Whitehouse PA, *et al.* The *ex vivo* characterization of XR5944 (MLN944) against a panel of human clinical tumor samples. Mol Cancer Ther 2004; 3(12): 1631-7.
[PMID: 15634657]

[72] Harris SM, Mistry P, Freathy C, Brown JL, Charlton PA. Antitumour activity of XR5944 *in vitro* and *in vivo* in combination with 5-fluorouracil and irinotecan in colon cancer cell lines. Br J Cancer 2005; 92(4): 722-8.
[http://dx.doi.org/10.1038/sj.bjc.6602403] [PMID: 15700035]

[73] Sappal DS, McClendon AK, Fleming JA, *et al.* Biological characterization of MLN944: A potent

DNA binding agent. Mol Cancer Ther 2004; 3(1): 47-58.
[PMID: 14749475]

[74]   Byers SA, Schafer B, Sappal DS, Brown J, Price DH. The antiproliferative agent MLN944 preferentially inhibits transcription. Mol Cancer Ther 2005; 4(8): 1260-7.
[http://dx.doi.org/10.1158/1535-7163.MCT-05-0109] [PMID: 16093442]

[75]   Verborg W, Thomas H, Bissett D, *et al.* First-into-man Phase I and pharmacokinetic study of XR5944.14, a novel agent with a unique mechanism of action. Br J Cancer 2007; 97(7): 844-50.
[http://dx.doi.org/10.1038/sj.bjc.6603953] [PMID: 17848959]

[76]   Punchihewa C, De Alba A, Sidell N, Yang D. XR5944: A potent inhibitor of estrogen receptors. Mol Cancer Ther 2007; 6(1): 213-9.
[http://dx.doi.org/10.1158/1535-7163.MCT-06-0392] [PMID: 17218634]

[77]   Moore MH, Hunter WN, d'Estaintot BL, Kennard O. DNA-drug interactions. The crystal structure of d(CGATCG) complexed with daunomycin. J Mol Biol 1989; 206(4): 693-705.
[http://dx.doi.org/10.1016/0022-2836(89)90577-9] [PMID: 2738914]

[78]   Pindur U, Haber M, Sattler K. Antitumor active drugs as intercalators of deoxyribonucleic acid: Molecular models of intercalation complexes. J Chem Educ 1993; 70: 263.
[http://dx.doi.org/10.1021/ed070p263]

[79]   Kim YS, Park SY, Lee HJ, Suh ME, Schollmeyer D, Lee CO. Synthesis and cytotoxicity of 6,11-dihydro-pyrido- and 6,11-dihydro-benzo[2,3-*b*]phenazine-6,11-dione derivatives. Bioorg Med Chem 2003; 11(8): 1709-14.
[http://dx.doi.org/10.1016/S0968-0896(03)00028-2] [PMID: 12659757]

[80]   Lee HJ, Kim JS, Park SY, *et al.* Synthesis and cytotoxicity evaluation of 6,11-dihydro-pyridazo- and 6,11-dihydro-pyrido[2,3-*b*]phenazine-6,11-diones. Bioorg Med Chem 2004; 12(7): 1623-8.
[http://dx.doi.org/10.1016/j.bmc.2004.01.029] [PMID: 15028255]

[81]   Lee HJ, Kim JS, Suh ME, *et al.* Synthesis and cytotoxicity evaluation of substituted pyridazino[4,5-*b*]phenazine-5,12-diones and tri/tetra-azabenzofluorene-5,6-diones. Eur J Med Chem 2007; 42(2): 168-74.
[http://dx.doi.org/10.1016/j.ejmech.2006.09.007] [PMID: 17070967]

[82]   Shaikh IA, Johnson F, Grollman AP. Streptonigrin. 1. Structure-activity relationships among simple bicyclic analogues. Rate dependence of DNA degradation on quinone reduction potential. J Med Chem 1986; 29(8): 1329-40.
[http://dx.doi.org/10.1021/jm00158a002] [PMID: 3525839]

[83]   Khalifa MMA, Ismail MMF, Noaman E. synthesis and *in vitro* cytotoxic activity of novel benzo [b] phenazine-6, 11-dione and 1, 4-naphthoquinone derivatives. Bull Pharm Sci 2008; 31: 69-80.

[84]   Cerecetto H, González M, Lavaggi ML, Azqueta A, López de Cerain A, Monge A. Phenazine 5,10-dioxide derivatives as hypoxic selective cytotoxins. J Med Chem 2005; 48(1): 21-3.
[http://dx.doi.org/10.1021/jm0492150] [PMID: 15633996]

[85]   Lavaggi ML, Cabrera M, González M, Cerecetto H. Differential enzymatic reductions governing the differential hypoxia-selective cytotoxicities of phenazine 5,10-dioxides. Chem Res Toxicol 2008; 21(9): 1900-6.
[http://dx.doi.org/10.1021/tx800199v] [PMID: 18661957]

[86]   Pachón OG, Azqueta A, Lavaggi ML, *et al.* Antitumoral effect of phenazine N^5,N^{10}-dioxide derivatives on Caco-2 cells. Chem Res Toxicol 2008; 21(8): 1578-85.
[http://dx.doi.org/10.1021/tx800032k] [PMID: 18553946]

[87]   Lavaggi ML, Cabrera M, Aravena MdeL, *et al.* Study of benzo[*a*]phenazine 7,12-dioxide as selective hypoxic cytotoxin-scaffold. Identification of aerobic-antitumoral activity through DNA fragmentation. Bioorg Med Chem 2010; 18(12): 4433-40.
[http://dx.doi.org/10.1016/j.bmc.2010.04.074] [PMID: 20471844]

[88]   Cerecetto H, González M, Lavaggi ML, *et al.* Phenazine 5,10-dioxide derivatives as hypoxic selective cytotoxins: Part II. Structure-activity relationship studies. Med Chem 2006; 2(5): 511-21.
[http://dx.doi.org/10.2174/157340606778250207] [PMID: 17017991]

[89]   Hanahan D, Weinberg RA. Hallmarks of cancer: The next generation. Cell 2011; 144(5): 646-74.
[http://dx.doi.org/10.1016/j.cell.2011.02.013] [PMID: 21376230]

[90]   Porporato PE, Dhup S, Dadhich RK, Copetti T, Sonveaux P. Anticancer targets in the glycolytic metabolism of tumors: A comprehensive review. Front Pharmacol 2011; 2: 49.
[http://dx.doi.org/10.3389/fphar.2011.00049] [PMID: 21904528]

[91]   Chowdhury G, Sarkar U, Pullen S, *et al.* DNA strand cleavage by the phenazine di-*N*-oxide natural product myxin under both aerobic and anaerobic conditions. Chem Res Toxicol 2012; 25(1): 197-206.
[http://dx.doi.org/10.1021/tx2004213] [PMID: 22084973]

[92]   Boulton AJ, Katritzky AR, Sewell MJ, Wallis B. *N*-oxides and related compounds. Part XXXI. The nuclear magnetic resonance spectra and tautomerism of some substituted benzofuroxans. J Chem Soc B 1967; 0: 914-9.
[http://dx.doi.org/10.1039/j29670000914]

[93]   Boulton AJ, Halls PJ, Katritzky AR. *N*-oxides ans related compounds. Part XXXVII. The effect of methyl and aza-substituents on the tautomeric equilibrium in benzofuroxan. J Chem Soc B 1970; 636-40.
[http://dx.doi.org/10.1039/j29700000636]

[94]   Cerecetto H, Gonzales M, Lavaggi ML, Porcal W. Benzofuroxan substituent effects in the preparation of N 5, N 10-dioxidevia expansion process with phenolates. J Braz Chem Soc 2005; 6: 1290-6.
[http://dx.doi.org/10.1590/S0103-50532005000700030]

[95]   Monge A, Palop JA, López de Ceráin A, *et al.* Hypoxia-selective agents derived from quinoxaline 1,4-di-N-oxides. J Med Chem 1995; 38(10): 1786-92.
[http://dx.doi.org/10.1021/jm00010a023] [PMID: 7752202]

[96]   Lavaggi ML, Cabrera M, Pintos C, *et al.* Novel phenazine 5,10-dioxides release •OH in simulated hypoxia and induce reduction of tumour volume *in vivo.* ISRN Pharmacol 2011; 1-11.

[97]   Lu Y, Li Y. Preparation of phenazine derivatives. CN106554321, 2017.

[98]   Gao X. Preparation of 2-chloro-N-(phenazin-2-yl)acetamide as anticancer agent. CN105418519, 2016.

[99]   Jiang F, Yan Y, Lu Y, *et al.* Preparation of pyrano[3, 2-α] phenazine derivatives useful as anticancer agents. CN105481869, 2016.

[100]   Feron O, Riant O, Kiss R, *et al.* Preparation of novel phenazine derivatives as antiangiogenic and anticancer agents. WO2012085222, 2012.

[101]   Camplo M, Siri O, Seillan C, *et al.* Derivatives of phenazines useful to treat cancer. WO2011117830, 2011.

[102]   Qian X, Yang P. Application of heterocyclic dinaphthalimide and its double- chained compound for treating tumor cells. CN1880313, 2006.

[103]   Takahata T, Sekimura N, Sumiyoshi Y. Preparation of quinoxalines and phenazines via benzofuroxans. JP2006241111, 2006.

[104]   Bigge CF, Elslager EF, French JC, *et al.* Antimicrobial and antitumor phenazine carboxaldehydes and derivatives. EP205339, 1986.

[105]   Medlen CE, Anderson R. Phenazine derivatives for treatment of cancer. ZA9208419, 1994.

[106]   Uda Y, Kumazawa Y, Nakagami Y, Amano T, Soda K, Sakakibara N. Preparation of 5-hydroxybenzo[a]phenazine-6-carboxylates as intermediates for antitumor agents. JP63083073, 1988.

[107]   Migita Y, Eguchi T, Kumazawa Y, *et al.* Benzo[a]phenazine derivatives, with antitumor activity, and a

process for their preparation. EP196910, 1986.

[108] Kim JS, Lee HJ, Suh ME. 6,11-dihydroquinoxalino[2,3-g]phthalazine-6,11-dione derivatives inhibiting cell growth and intermediates and process for preparing them. KR2005017866, 2005.

[109] Mao Z, Zheng X, Tan C, Huang H, Ji L. Organic hybrid tetranuclear Pt complex, preparation method and application in preparing antitumor medicine thereof. WO2012155559, 2012.

[110] Døskeland SO, Rongved P, Herfindal L, *et al.* Compounds. WO2015063516, 2015.

[111] Rongved P, Aastrand OAH, Viktorsson E O, Samuelson O, Heikal A. Preparation of N-oxide heterocycles for use in the treatment of cancer and bacterial diseases. WO2018109504, 2018.

[112] Li Y, Rong H, Zhao L, Xu L. Manufacture of novel phenazine antitumor antibiotic with *Streptomyces*. CN103993050, 2014.

[113] Ju J, Song Y, Huang H, Zhang Y. A phenazine compounds and its application in producing anticancer medicines. CN103360329, 2013.

[114] Lu Y, Yan Y, Wang L, *et al.* Design, facile synthesis and biological evaluations of novel pyrano[3,2-a]phenazine hybrid molecules as antitumor agents. Eur J Med Chem 2017; 127: 928-43.
[http://dx.doi.org/10.1016/j.ejmech.2016.10.068] [PMID: 27836197]

CHAPTER 4

Cancer Stem Cell Targeting For Anticancer Therapy: Strategies and Challenges

Sanjoy Das[1], Malay K. Das[1,*] and Tapash Chakraborty[2]

[1] *Department of Pharmaceutical Sciences, Dibrugarh University, Dibrugarh, Assam, 786004, India*

[2] *Girijananda Chowdhury Institute of Pharmaceutical Science, Hatkhowapara, Azara, Guwahati, Assam, 781017, India*

Abstract: Cancer Stem Cells (CSCs) are those tumour cells, which possess the ability to self-renew, form a new tumour, produce progeny of multiple phenotypes and are responsible for maintaining the growth of the tumour. CSCs have different gene expressions and signalling pathways compared to other tumour cells. The mutation in the CSC gene is the main reason for cancer initiation, progression, metastasis, recurrence and drug resistance. Hence, targeting the CSCs selectively can cure the disease without much damage to the healthy tissues caused by traditional chemotherapy and radiotherapy. Previous works have shown various therapeutic strategies for cancer using new drugs molecules, nanomedicines, specific surface markers of CSCs, modulators of signalling pathways, agents for adjustment of the microenvironment signals, drug-efflux pump inhibitors, manipulators of miRNA expression, inducers of CSCs apoptosis and differentiation. A few selective novel compounds and therapeutic strategies targeting CSCs are presently in preclinical and clinical trials. This chapter highlights the novel strategies targeting CSCs for the successful treatment of cancer. The challenges in the development of new strategies leading to the eradication of cancer and recent patents issued in the area of CSCs targeting are also discussed.

Keywords: Acute myeloid leukaemia, apoptosis, brain cancer stem cells, cancer, breast cancer resistance protein, cancer stem cells, chemoresistance, DNA damage response, glioma stem cells, gold nanoparticles, insulin potentiated therapy, mesoporous silica nanoparticles, metastasis, *mi*RNA, nanomedicine, P-glycoprotein, signalling pathways, *si*RNA, surface markers, targeted anticancer therapy.

* **Corresponding author Malay K. Das:** Department of Pharmaceutical Sciences, Dibrugarh University, Dibrugarh, Assam, 786004, India; Tel: +91-9954229317; E-mail: mkdps@dibru.ac.in

Atta-ur-Rahman and Khurshid Zaman (Eds.)

1. INTRODUCTION

The body tissues are generally derived from organ-specific Stem Cells (SCs), which take part in normal tissue growth and renewal. The unique properties of SCs like self- renewability, pluripotency, differentiability and the ability to remain dormant for long durations (Fig. **1**) make them easily distinguishable from the rest of the cells. When a stem cell is divided, it generates two daughter cells - one persists a stem cell and the other one becomes a transit-amplifying cell, leading the mechanism of differentiation [1, 2]. The mutations in the genetic materials of SCs may be the reason for the formation of Cancer Stem Cells (CSCs) [3, 4]. The CSCs are neoplastic cells with distinct survival mechanisms and stem cell properties essential for the maintenance and propagation of the tumour. In the growth of cancer, some CSCs do not actively proliferate but serve as reserve populations [5, 6]. The renewal of normal cells by cell division in normal tissues and further differentiation do not increase the number of cells in the tissues [7, 8]. The number of stem cells in cancer increases with time because the transit-amplifying cells either resume to proliferate and do not mature or the mature cells do not die or both occur simultaneously [9]. The CSCs have the capability to generate new tumorigenic cells by self-renewal process as well as undergo differentiation to produce phenotypically diverse non-tumorigenic cells [10, 11].

Though the concept of CSCs was recognized over several decades ago, the identification and characterization of CSCs in haematological malignancies and many other types of cancers were made possible only in the last two decades [12, 13]. The concept that cancers originate from stem cells has evolved over the last 200 years and was first formulated as the embryonal rest theory of cancer in the mid-1800s [14]. The embryonic rest theory proposes that cancer generates from a small collection of embryonic tissues, which persists and does not undergo differentiation into mature tissues [15]. However, the embryonal rest theory of cancer was disregarded during the last half of the 19th century due to the lack of further experimental support and was replaced by the de-differentiation theory of cancer [16]. The de-differentiation theory of cancer suggests that cancers derive from fully grown differentiated cells through de-differentiation, which exhibit the properties of CSCs [17].

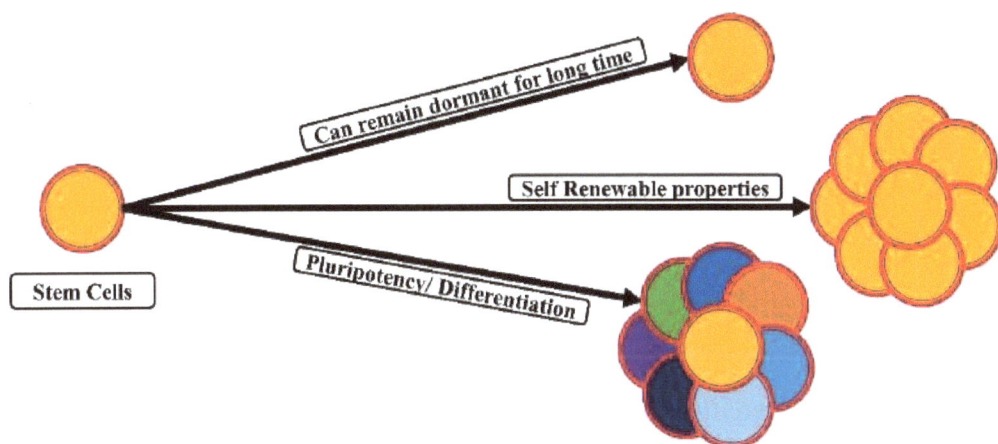

Fig. (1). Unique properties of stem cells that make them different from other normal cells.

The CSCs are hypothesized to originate from tumour progenitor cells or dedifferentiated cells that acquire the characteristics of CSCs [18, 19]. The hypothesis of CSCs is mainly based on two separate, but related components. The first one concerns the cellular origin of cancer i.e. cancer arises from the stem cells and the second one concerns the cellular components of cancer i.e. the cancer is composed of the same type of cells like normal tissues [20, 21]. As reported by the accepted hypothesis of CSCs, the malignant transformation indicates the presence of a cell population with definite properties like self-healing ability [22]. The self-healing capability of CSCs is adequate to trigger or sustain the malignant progression leading to heterogeneous tumours. Almost all cancer types are composed of heterogeneous cell populations [23, 24]. These cell populations constitute the critical subset within the tumour mass, which conserves the tumour and leads to the aggressive nature of the tumour [25]. Throughout the progression of cancer, CSCs can additionally be generated from differentiated cancer cells via adaptation within the tumour microenvironment along with responses from therapeutic pressures and consequent generation of heterogeneous phenotypes [26, 27]. The functional and phenotypic heterogeneity are the most admissible properties of CSCs within many tumour types with inter-tumour and intra-tumour complexity [28]. The inter-tumour heterogeneity can be found in tumours of the same tissue type found in different patients, while intra-tumour heterogeneity can be observed in tumours within a single patient [29].

The genomic landscape of individual tumours and their clonal evolution, the existence of different populations of cancer cells with CSCs residing at the top of the hierarchy and the influence of the tumour microenvironment have been suggested as the reasons for the inter-tumoural and inter-tumoural heterogeneities

[30 - 32]. Generally, there are two controversial models describing the heterogeneity in tumours such as CSC model and the stochastic model [33]. The CSC model, known as a hierarchical model, suggests that the growth and progression of many cancers are driven by small, but distinctive subpopulations of CSCs; while the stochastic model or evolution model predicts that a tumour is biologically homogeneous and the behaviour of the cancer cells is randomly influenced by unpredicted intrinsic and/or extrinsic factors [34]. Both stochastic and hierarchical models have been hypothesized to describe tumour heterogeneity, but alone each model is insufficient to explain the diversity within tumours [35]. Moreover, the heterogeneity of CSCs is mainly regulated by intrinsic and extrinsic differences [36]. The intrinsic differences include genetic mutations and epigenetic changes that contribute to tumour heterogeneity; whereas extrinsic differences are considered to be surrounding microenvironmental factors like cell to cell interactions, various chemotactic factors, cytokine concentrations and hypoxic conditions that interact with cancer cells to aid its progression [37]. The advanced sequencing techniques and epigenetic research have also clarified that the genetic modification of CSCs is responsible for CSC heterogeneity i.e., instability of CSCs genome includes chromosomal instability with frequent mutation [38]. At the same time, CSCs undergo clonal evaluation leading to generate new subclones. These subclones of CSCs along with numerous molecular functions and adaptable genetic mutations exhibit the dominant stem cell population and contribute to tumour progression or malignant transformation [39 - 41]. Moreover, CSCs possess a highly efficient DNA damage response (DDR) system, which is considered as a promoter to the resistance of these cells from exposure to DNA damaging agents [42]. Although DDR is critical to the preservation of genome stability, highly efficient DNA repair machinery of CSCs can reduce the efficacy of DNA damaging agents in treating cancers [43].

The CSCs often exhibit a high number of genes involved in pro-survival signalling and drug-efflux mechanisms [44]. The signalling pathways such as Wnt/β-catenin, Notch, Hedgehog, Transforming Growth Factor (TGF-β)/Bone Morphogenetic Proteins (BMP), Epidermal Growth Factor Receptor (EGFR)/Mitogen-Activated Protein Kinase (MAPK) and Nuclear Factor-kappa activated B cells (NF-κB)/Signal Transducer and Activator of Transcription 3 (STAT3) pathways regulate the self-renewal and differentiation of normal stem cells. These pathways are normally deregulated in CSCs with stem cell phenotype [45 - 47]. Deregulation of these signalling pathways is normally connected to an Epithelial-Mesenchymal Transition (EMT) and such signalling pathways are mediated by microRNA (*mi*RNA) and EMT-inducing transcription factors [48, 49], imparting self-renewal potential to CSCs [50].

The self-renewal, tumour heterogeneity, tumour plasticity and multilineage differentiation capability of CSCs are believed to stimulate initiation and growth of the tumour, generating the full repository of cancer cells [51, 52]. The first CSCs were identified in the bone marrow of Acute Myeloid Leukaemia (AML) patients in 1997 [53]. Subsequently, the CSCs have been identified and characterized in many cancers including hematologic malignancies and solid tumours e.g. breast cancer, brain tumours, pancreatic cancer, colon cancer, liver cancer, lung cancer, ovarian cancer, malignant melanoma and prostate cancer [54 - 56]. The identification and characterization of CSCs are mainly dependent on a surface marker shared with normal stem cells. The CSC surface markers have been identified or isolated in multiple types of cancers including acute myeloid leukaemia [57], breast cancer [58], brain cancer [59], multiple myeloma [60], pancreatic cancer [61], head and neck squamous cell carcinoma [62], colon cancer [63], liver cancer [64], lung cancer [65], ovarian cancer [66] and prostate cancer [67]. Clinical and preclinical studies revealed that adult stem cells could transform into CSCs with specific types of surface markers. The targeting of these specific surface markers on CSCs has been desired to be a good alternative for cancer treatment [68]. The types of surface markers carried by different types of cancers are listed in Table **1** [69 - 101].

Table 1. Cell Surface Markers Present on CSCs.

Cancer Type	Surface Markers	Reference(s)
Bladder cancer	$CD44^+/CK5^+/CK20^-$, $CD44^+/CD44v6^+/EMA^-$, $67LR^{+(bright)}/CD66c^{-(dim)}/K17^+$, $CD133^+/Oct3/4^+/Nestin^+$, Keratin 14 $(KRT14)^+$	[69, 70]
Brain cancer	$BCRP1^+$, $SSEA-1^+$, $CD133^+/CD44^+/Nestin^+$, $CD133^+/CXCR4^+$ $CD133^+$, $HMOX1^+$, $CD97^+$, $CD15^+$, $A2B5^+/CD133^-$, Integrin $\alpha6^-$, $L1CAM^+/CD133^+$	[71]
Breast cancer	ESA^+, $CD44^+$, $CD24^{-/low}$, $Lineage^-$, $ALDH-1^{high}$, $ALDH1^+/CD44^+/CD24^{-/low}$, $CD44^+/CD24^{-/low}/EpCAM^+$, $CD44^+/CD49f^{high}/CD133/2^{high}$	[72]
Colon cancer	$CD133^+$, $CD44^+$, $CD166^+$, $EpCAM^+$, $CD24^+$	[73]
Colorectal cancer	ESA^+, $ALDH^{high}$, $CD133^+/CD44^+/ALDH1^+$, $EpCAM^+/CD44^+/CD166^-$, $CD44^+/CD24^+$, $CD133^+/CD24^+$, $Lgr5^+$	[74, 75]
Gastric cancer	$CD44^+$, $Lgr5^+$, $CD133^-$, $EpCAM^+/CD44^+$, $CD44^+/CD24^+$, $CD44^+/CD54^+$, $CD90^+$	[76]
Gallbladder cancer	$CD44^+/CD133^+$, $EpCAM^-/CD44^+/CD13^+$, $CD133^+$	[77, 78]
Head and neck cancer	$CD44^+$, $CD24^+$	[79]
Kidney cancer	$CD105^+$, $CD133^+$, $CD44^+/CD24^-$	[80]
Acute myeloid leukaemia	$CD34^+$, $CD38^-$, $HLA-DR-CD71^-$, $CD90^-$, $CD117^-$, $CD123^+$, $CD47^+$, $CCL-1^+$, $CD96^+$, $TIM3^+$, $CD32^-$, $CD25^+$	[81, 82]

(Table 1) contd.....

Cancer Type	Surface Markers	Reference(s)
Liver cancer	ESA⁺, CD133⁺/CD49f⁺, CD90⁺/CD45⁻, CD13⁺, EpCAM⁺, CD44⁺/CD133⁺, CD44⁺/CD90⁺, SALL4⁺/EpCAM+	[83, 84]
Lung cancer	CD133⁺, CD44⁺, ALDH1⁺, CD117⁺, ABCG2^{high}	[85]
Melanoma	ABCB5⁺, CD133⁺, CD271⁺, CD20⁺, CXCR6⁻, JARID1B⁺	[86, 87]
Multiple myeloma	CD138⁻	[88, 89]
Esophageal cancer	Integrin α7⁺, CD44⁺/ALDH1⁺	[90, 91]
Ovarian cancer	CD133⁺, ALDH1⁺, CD44⁺, CD117⁺	[92, 93]
Pancreatic cancer	ESA⁺, CD133⁺, CD44⁺, EpCAM⁺, CD24⁺	[94, 95]
Prostate cancer	CD44⁺, α2β1^{high}, CD133⁺, ALDH^{high}, PSA$^{-/low}$	[96, 97]
Sarcoma	CD29⁺/CD133⁺/Nestin⁺, CD133⁺, CD133⁺/Nestin⁺, CD117⁺/Stro-1⁺	[98, 99]
Thyroid cancer	ALDH1⁺, CD133⁺, CD44⁺/CD24⁻, SEEA1⁺	[100]
Uterine cancer	ALDH1⁺/CD126⁺, CD133⁺	[101]

The CSCs are the main reasons for therapeutic failure against cancer and can trigger the repopulation of tumour growth post-therapy [102]. The CSCs are also resistant to medical therapy and contribute to high rates of tumour reoccurrence or relapse [103]. These cells can be either intrinsically resistant to therapy and cause a relapse or extrinsically instructed by the tumour microenvironment to become resistant under the selective pressure of therapy [104]. The therapeutic failure in cancer generally occurs due to the fact that the conventional therapies target only the bulk of the tumour and are unable to target CSCs due to their high resistance in nature, leading to metastasis and recurrence of the tumour [105 - 107]. Modern cancer theory often faces challenges in the identification and targeting of neoplastic stem cells even after successful initial therapy and recovery [108]. The various types of intrinsic and extrinsic factors are significantly responsible for controlling the progression of the cell cycle in CSCs, including differentiation, tumour cellular plasticity, multidrug resistance and signal transduction. In order to develop more effective approaches for cancer treatment, a new generation of cancer therapeutics has been designed or developed for complete removal of CSCs by interfering with the pathways mentioned above [109 - 111]. Researchers are trying to develop new molecular therapies specifically directed against these cells. Such molecular therapies against CSCs are reported to be more effective as they induce tumour regression by reducing the occurrence of new cancer cells [112, 113]. Therefore, the development of specific targeted therapies against CSCs may potentially prevent tumour recurrence and hold great promises for improving the survival rate of cancer patients (Fig. **2**).

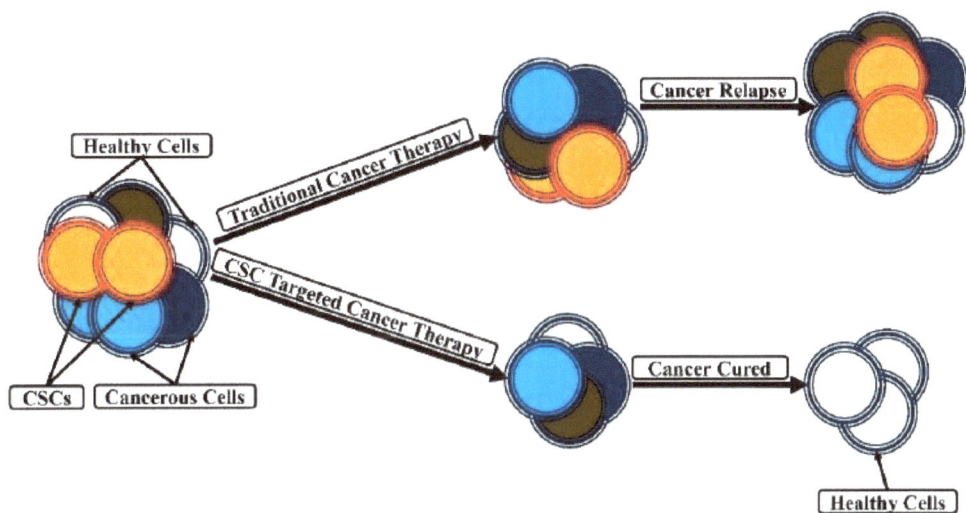

Fig. (2). Difference between traditional and CSC targeted anticancer therapy.

2. CURRENT STRATEGIES TARGETING CSCS

The research for identification and isolation of CSCs has just been started and a long way is yet to go before we have a robust system. Though the recent studies have identified various CSC surface antigens, the picture is not clear. It is seen that the CSCs of different types of cancers do not express the same markers, or some normal cells also possess these surface antigens [114]. Therefore, absolute isolation of CSCs is yet not possible, but commonly believed that CSCs are prospectively isolated using methods based on either a surface marker or an intracellular enzyme activity [115]. Moreover, identification of CSCs must be based on the ability of the cells to form spheres in serum-free medium (or in agar medium) and to initiate tumour growth after serial transplantation in immune-compromised animal models [116 - 118]. However, these techniques also have their own limitations. The *in vitro* assay may not detect active stem cells that are incapable of developing spheres due to the lack of additional extrinsic signals needed for their activation. Since a considerable number of cells are required to induce tumour growth *in vivo*, due to insertion in a foreign microenvironment deficient in specific signals for survival and development, serial transplantation technique may fail as the number of CSCs present on the samples may be very low [119]. Therefore, to address CSCs specifically in further experiments, it is necessary to isolate cells based on surface markers and subsequently to assess their functional abilities by specific *in vitro* and *in vivo* assays [120].

Chemotherapy, surgery and radiotherapy are commonly used therapies against various types of cancers like breast cancer [121], metastatic brain tumours [122], lung cancer [123], ovarian cancer [124], and colorectal cancer [125]. Chemotherapy targets cells that grow and divide quickly, as cancer cells. Unlike radiotherapy or surgery, which targets specific areas, chemotherapy can work throughout the whole body leading to affects various fast-growing healthy tissues like skin, hair, intestine and bone marrow [126 - 128]. These therapies have multiple and serious limitations, because the agents do not kill cancer cells selectively and affect the healthy cells as well, resulting in treatment failure and cancer recurrence [129]. The chemotherapeutic agents mostly target the rapidly dividing cells, but CSCs may remain undivided for prolonged periods [130]. Moreover, the CSC possesses a high expression of drug-efflux pumps, high capacity for DNA repairing and resistance to micro-environmental characteristics like hypoxia and acidosis [131]. Thus, the elimination of CSCs is not easy and hence targeting the CSCs becomes essential in treating cancer and preventing tumour relapse [132, 133].

Researchers have developed different strategies to target the CSCs and their cell colonies as represented in Fig. (**3**). These include new drugs molecules, targeted nanocarriers by targeting specific surface markers, modulation of signalling pathways, adjustment of the micro-environmental signals, inhibition of the drug-efflux pumps of CSCs, manipulation of *mi*RNA expression, induction of CSCs apoptosis and differentiation.

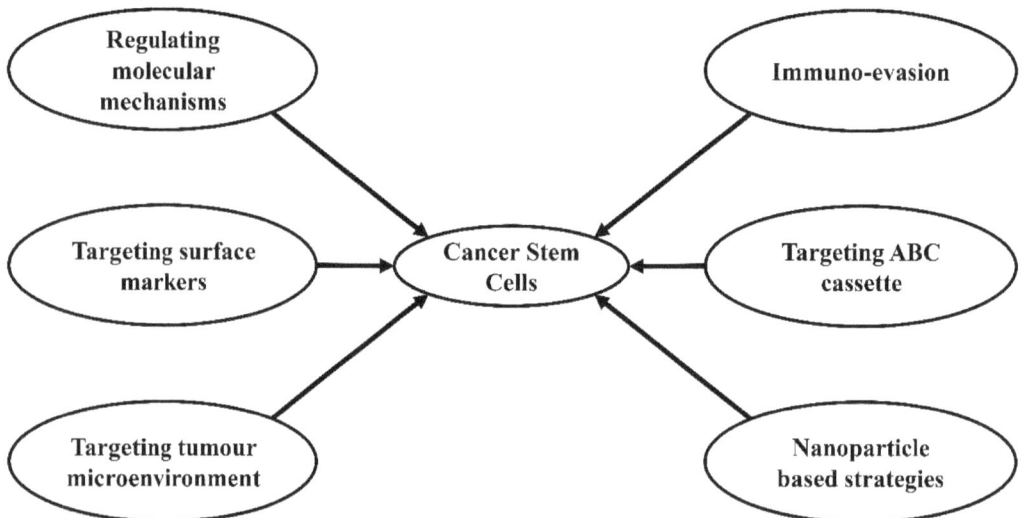

Fig. (3). Novel therapeutic strategies for targeting cancer stem cells.

2.1. CSC-Specific Chemotherapeutic Agents to Overcome Drug Resistance

2.1.1. Synthetic CSC Targeted Drug Molecules

The conventional chemotherapeutic agents kill the cells of a growing tumour without any discrimination to the types of cells present in them [134]. However, as discussed earlier, the CSCs present within the tumours are more resistant to the therapeutic agents than the other tumour cells. These survived CSCs again relapse the tumour attached to the patients. Researchers have shown that some drugs or a combination of drugs not only eliminates the tumour cells, but also eliminates all the cancer cells (CSCs and non-CSCs) at once [135]. Hence, they reduce the chances of tumour relapse completely. These therapeutic agents eliminate the CSCs by different mechanisms (Table **2**). Moreover, cancer risk is reduced in patients with diabetes who receive metformin [136]. The anticancer efficacy of metformin has attained growing interest due to its inhibitory effects on CSCs. The anticancer mechanism of metformin is based on suppression of oncogenic signalling pathways, receptor tyrosine kinase, Phosphatidylinositol 3-Kinase (PI3K/Akt) and mammalian Target Of Rapamycin (mTOR) pathways [137]. Additionally, metformin also inhibits CSC sphere-forming *in vitro* as well as *in vivo* xenografts and excites many cancers like breast cancer, pancreatic cancer, colon cancer and glioma [138]. Notably, the presence of efflux pumps on the cell membrane of the CSC is an important mechanism of drug resistance [139]. In CSCs, the higher expression of ATP-Binding Cassette (ABC) transporters can be identified by treatment with Hoechst 33342 dye [140]. Dye efflux assays using fluorophores by flow cytometry are used to determine the presence of these transporters in specific cell populations [141]. Numerous pharmacological moieties including P-glycoprotein (P-gp) inhibitors, nanomedicines, Tyrosine Kinase Inhibitors (TKIs), small interfering RNA (*si*RNA) and *mi*RNA that can be interacting with ABC transporters superfamily have been demonstrated to inhibit the multidrug resistance [142, 143]. Researchers have developed/identified drugs that can decrease either the expression or the functions of ABC transporters. The first generation modulators or inhibitors of ABC transporters include molecules such as Verapamil, Quinine and Cyclosporine-A [144]. In preclinical studies, they showed good results, but in clinical trials, few beneficial effects were observed [145]. To overcome the limitations of the first generation modulators of ABC transporters and to have better efficacy, drugs like Valspodar (PSC-833) and Ebiricodar (VX710) have been developed. They are the second generation modulators of ABC transporters. They showed better efficacy than the first generation modulators when used in combination with traditional chemotherapy. However, they showed some serious adverse effects on hepatic and intestinal metabolism by inhibiting the enzymes of the cytochrome P450 family and reducing the clearance of the drug [146]. The third generation modulators of ABC transporters, such as Elacridar (GF120918), Zosuquidar (LY335979) and Tariquidar (XR9576), have also been developed and are more active with fewer side effects compared to first and second generation modulators [147].

Table 2. List of Chemotherapeutic Agents Used for Targeting CSCs According to their Mechanism of Actions.

Chemotherapeutic Agents	Mechanism of Actions
ABC transporters- • The first generation modulators - Verapamil (P-gp inhibitor), Quinine and Cyclosporine-A, CDF, ALDHs, DEAB • The second-generation modulators - Valspodar (PSC-833) and Ebiricodar (VX710) • The third generation modulators - Elacridar (GF120918), Zosuquidar (LY335979), Tariquidar (XR9576) Natural agents- • EGCG, Curcumin, Berberine, Isoliquiritigenin	Overcome drug resistance in CSCs
• DC-cell vaccine (ALDH^{bright} antigen) • T-cell vaccine (ASB4 antigen) • Nivolumab (PD-1 immune checkpoint inhibitors)	Targeting immune cells in CSC
• H90 (anti-CD44) • P245 (anti-CD44) • H4C4 (anti-CD44) • GV5 (anti-CD44R1) • RO5429083 (anti-CD44, targets a glycosylated extracellular constant domain of CD44) • BsAb (anti-CD3/anti-CD133) Nanocarriers- • Doxorubicin loaded liposomes conjugated with anti-CD44 antibody to specifically target the CD44-positive hepatocellular carcinoma • Salinomycin loaded nanocarriers conjugated with CD133 aptamers to selectively inhibit CD133$^+$ osteosarcoma	Targeting cell surface markers in CSCs
• The Wnt/β catenin pathway - Dkk1, *si*RNA, XAV939 • The notch pathway - γ-secretase inhibitors, DLL inhibitors, mAbs (Demcizumab) • TGFβ/BMP - SMAD 6/SMAD7 • The hedgehog pathway - Cyclopamine, Vismodegib (GDC-0449), IPI269609 Nanocarriers- • Curcumin-loaded PLGA nanocarriers suppress Wnt/β-catenin signalling • Polyethyleneimine/PEG-conjugated MSNPs loaded with LY364947	Targeting signalling pathways in CSCs
• AMD3100 • NOX-A12 • Fruquintinib (HMPL-013)	Affecting the microenvironment signals in CSCs

(Table 2) contd.....

Chemotherapeutic Agents	Mechanism of Actions
• Sunitinib (chemosensitivity modulated by *mi*R-21) • Demethoxycurcumin (chemosensitivity modulated by *mi*R-145)	Modulation of miRNA expression in CSCs
• Cisplatin and Bortezomib (TRAIL combination therapy) • Parthenolide, Pyrrolidine-dithiocarbamate (NF-κB inhibitors)	Induction of apoptosis in CSCs
• Bevacizumab • Sunitinib, Pazopanib, Sorafenib and Fruquintinib (HMPL-013) • Oncothyreon, Topotecan and Digoxin (target the HIF pathway)	Targeting CSC niches

2.1.2. Natural CSC Targeted Drug Molecules

Researchers have investigated some natural modulators of ABC transporters to treat multidrug-resistant cancers. These natural modulators of ABC transporters have a synergistic effect with other anti-tumour drugs. These natural modulators compete for the active sites of efflux pumps and thus reduce the chemotherapeutic efflux [148]. Among the natural modulators, flavonoids stand out as efflux pump inhibitors as they interact with the ATP-binding sites by inhibiting the ATPase activity of P-gp [149, 150]. For example, Epigallocatechin-3-Gallate (EGCG), an active phenolic compound of green tea exhibits antitumor properties [151]. EGCG decreased the activity and expression of ABCB1/P-gp and ABCG2/Breast Cancer Resistance Protein (BCRP) genes in Tamoxifen-resistant breast cancer cells [152]. Structural studies have shown that the EGCG binds to the ATP-binding site of the ABCB1/P-gp transporter [153].

Curcuma longa is the biological source of Curcumin, another most potent and studied polyphenols. Researchers have shown that the combination of curcumin with other anticancer agents, such as Tamoxifen, Cisplatin, Doxorubicin and Vincristine, can effectively eliminate cancer cells *in vitro* [154 - 158]. Similarly, another flavonoid apigenin, present in various vegetables and medicinal plants has also been reported to possess anti-mutagenic properties [159, 160]. Moreover, the isoquinoline alkaloid berberine shows therapeutic potential against several disorders [161 - 163]. It has been reported to reduce the expression of genes related to the pluripotency of stem cells and decrease the percentage of side populations in the pancreatic tumour cells [164]. Berberine was reported to reduce the expression of ABCC1/Multidrug Resistance Protein (MPR) and ABCG2/BCRP genes in human breast cancer cells [165]. Isoliquiritigenin, a phenolic chemical compound found in liquorice has been reported to possess anti-proliferative, metastasis suppressive and angiogenesis properties [166, 167]. Isoliquiritigenin is a chemo-sensitizer that exhibits synergistic effects with common anticancer drugs like 5-Fluorouracil, Epirubicin and Taxol, mainly in breast cancer cell lines. In *in vitro* studies, it reduced the cancer cell population in the presence or absence of Epirubicin in the breast cancer cell lines [168].

2.1.3. Insulin Potentiated Chemotherapy as an Alternative Therapeutic Strategy for CSCs

Insulin Potentiated Therapy (IPT) can also be considered as a novel therapeutic strategy in CSCs targeting. The IPT is a controversial alternative to cancer treatment utilizing insulin as a supplement to low-dose chemotherapy. The recognized physiological action of insulin is increasing the cell membrane permeability so that anticancer drugs are absorbed faster into cancerous cells improving pharmacological actions of medications administered jointly in the therapy [169]. Simultaneously, an excessive number of insulin receptors are also found on the surface of CSCs such as insulin-like growth factor I and II (IGF-I and IGF-II), Tyrosine Kinase Receptors (TKRs) and Insulin Receptors (IRs) [170, 171]. These receptors transmit various signalling pathways like the PI3K/Akt pathway and MAPK pathway, which plays a vital role in human malignancies and cancer progression [172]. Hence, blocking these signalling pathways is a promising strategy to selectively inhibit the tumour promoting effects. Accordingly, giving insulin just before the infusion of low dose chemotherapeutic agents, generally in a combined form to interrupt several sites of the cell cycle, induces minimum adverse effects and arrests the cancer cells suspiciously to reconstruct an efficient immune response [173].

2.1.4. Combination Therapy Against CSCs

Considering the transformation of cancer cells to CSCs, it is broadly accepted that both cancer cells and CSCs must be eliminated to improve the therapeutic efficacy of anticancer drugs [174]. Both chemotherapy and CSCs-specific therapy alone are inadequate to cure cancer. Thus the search for an alternative therapy specific for CSCs-targeting is needed [175]. The combined therapy comprising conventional chemotherapeutics with an anti-CSC agent could offer a promising strategy for eliminating both cancer cells and CSCs [176]. Researchers have found that Salinomycin is a promising CSCs-targeting agent as it particularly suppresses cancer stem-like cells in several cancer types with diverse mechanisms like the blockade of EMT process, triggering of apoptosis, interference of the Wnt/β-catenin signalling pathway, inhibition of ABC transporters [177, 178]. In contrast, conventional chemotherapeutics like Paclitaxel exhibit a nominal effect on the growth and proliferation of breast CSCs. Therefore, the combination of Salinomycin with Paclitaxel is a promising combined therapy to improve tumour cell killing [179]. Furthermore, Salinomycin combined with Gemcitabine eliminates pancreatic cancer cells. Salinomycin suppresses the progression of CSCs, while Gemcitabine inhibits the growth of non-CSCs. Customarily *in vivo* studies revealed that Salinomycin combined with Gemcitabine could eradicate the engrossment of human pancreatic cancer more efficiently than the individual agents [180]. Apart from the above outstanding benefits, combined therapy has numerous shortcomings that may lead to treatment failure due to the fact that drug synergism cannot be assured, attainment of the optimal synergistic drug ratio is challenging and uptake of the drug into the tumour cell is inconsistent. Nanomedicines can be a safe, potent and effective form of drug delivery carrier, which may resolve the problems allied with combination chemotherapy. Therefore, Salinomycin-loaded Nanoparticles (NPs) combined with Gefitinib-loaded NPs were developed and results showed that such a combined platform represent a potential approach for lung cancer by inhibiting both lung CSCs and cancer cells [181, 182].

2.2. Immunotherapy or Vaccination Therapy Against CSCs

In order to improve the CSC-specific therapies by targeted small molecule inhibitors, the commencement of immunotherapy has led to inspiring developments in employing CSC specific antigen offering to control the power of the body immune system to improve cancer therapies [183]. Immunotherapy targets CSCs by body immune cells, like Cytokine-Induced Killer (CIK) cells, Natural Killer (NK) cells, Dendritic Cells (DCs), Gamma delta T (γδ T) cells and CD8+ T-cells or Cytotoxic T Lymphocytes (CTLs) [184]. The CIK cells are a class of immune effector cells highlighting a combined T-cell and NK cell similar phenotype. The CIK cells inducing apoptosis in tumour cells is due to the secretion of numerous cytokines including Interleukin-2 (IL-2) and Interferon-gamma (IFN-γ), regulating the body's immune system [185, 186]. The NK cells are major effector cells for innate immunity enriched with essential cytolytic functions [187]. Certain CSCs have been susceptible to expressing NK cell-specific ligands like Nectin-2 and poliovirus receptor-mediated protein that force their exposure to IL-2 as well as IL-15 activated NK cell killing [188]. Moreover, CIK cells, NK cells and activated T cells with overexpressing Programmed cell Death 1 (PD-1)/ Programmed cell Death Ligand (PD-L1) immune checkpoints, are involved in tumour immune-evasion in a wide variety of malignant cells. Thus, exploring new agents or combinational approaches that block such immune checkpoints is a hopeful strategy to enhance antitumor effects [189]. The most effective antigen offering DCs in a human body presents tumour antigens to T lymphocytes inducing antitumor immune responses [190]. The DCs pulsed with CSC lysates or cancer cell lines have been utilized as vaccines to investigate the therapeutic outcome by inducing IL-4 and IFN-γ secretion in vaccinated mice and results suggest the suppression of tumour progression and prolonged survival of immunized mice [191]. Another important antigen source of DCs is Aldehyde Dehydrogenase (ALDH)[bright], a reliable CSC marker in the D5 and the SCC7 murine tumour models. To test the immunogenicity, DCs pulsed with tumour-derived ALDH[bright] cells were vaccinated 2-3 times into mice earlier to challenge with syngeneic tumours and results suggested that DCs pulsed with ALDH[bright] cells significantly inhibit the tumour growth [192]. Moreover, γδ T cells, which also do not need Major Histocompatibility Complex (MHC) presentation for activation, have been studied for their ability to target CSCs and consequently upregulate CD54 and MHC1 on CSCs, which results in consecutive sensitization to CD8+ T cells targeting the CSCs at numerous stages of differentiation that may obtain outstanding results in various cancers [193]. The ASB4, an antigen specific to CSCs, has been found particularly in a subset of CSCs in colonic cancer and the adoptively transported CTLs particular for ASB4 are able to selectively kill the CSCs of colonic cancer. Thus, CTL-based vaccination or immunotherapies toward colonic CSCs might be a promising strategy for its complete eradication [194]. Therefore targeting CSCs through immune cell vaccines may foster the development of novel CSC-targeted immunological therapeutics for cancer treatment.

2.3. CSC-Targeted Nanocarriers for Chemotherapeutic Agents

Nanocarrier-based therapeutic approaches provide advantages over the small molecular pharmaceutical agents based therapeutic strategies [195]. The ideal nanocarriers should specifically target the diseased tissues, which minimizes or avoids off-target effects of the active therapeutic agents on healthy tissues [196]. This strategy involves the conjugation of several types of targeting ligands to the surface of NPs that are specific to the diseased cell surface components and are unique to pathological tissues. These targeting ligands may be small molecules, polypeptide-based peptides, protein domains, antibodies and nucleic acid-based aptamers [197]. Ligands from multiple classes or multiple ligands within the same class but with different targets (multi-valency and multi-specificity) have been implemented to enhance nanocarrier targeting. Each ligand class has particular advantages, disadvantages, unique attributes and conjugation strategies [198]. However, this powerful technology leads to a decreased toxicity in non-targeted cells and thus improves the distribution of nanomaterials in the target cells [199]. A wide variety of long blood circulating nanomaterials like carbon-based (e.g., nanodiamond), metal-based (e.g., gold and silver NPs), lipid-based (liposomes), quantum dots, magnetic and polymeric NPs have been developed with various sizes and modifications to their surfaces with ligand(s) for enhancing the drug targeting efficacy in CSCs [200 - 202]. All these NPs mentioned above have their unique properties, such as high surface to volume ratio, easiness to be modified, unique optical properties, quantum-size effects [203]. Taking advantage of these outstanding properties of various nanocarriers will further contribute to obtaining better solutions for targeted and controlled eradication of CSCs in the future.

2.3.1. Targeting CSC-Specific Markers

A cluster of Differentiation (CD) 44 is a transmembrane receptor for hyaluronic acid and has been reported to be present in CSCs from numerous solid tumours, including breast, bladder, cervical, colon, gastric, lung, ovarian, pancreatic and prostate cancers (Table **1**). Various nanocarriers have been reported to target the CD44 surface markers of the CSCs successfully *in vitro.* Paclitaxel-loaded micelles have been shown to remarkably increase the therapeutic efficacy and specificity in CD44-positive metastatic ovarian cancer cells isolated from patients [204]. An anti-CD44 antibody-incorporated liposome loaded with doxorubicin has been reported to specifically target the CD44-positive hepatocellular carcinoma cells and effectively induce apoptosis [205]. Though several nanocarriers have been demonstrated to target CD44$^+$ cells *in vitro*, their therapeutic effects *in vivo* have not yet been studied due to non-specificity of CD44 found in both normal stem cells and CSCs. Moreover, targeting CD44 using monoclonal antibodies arrives a tolerable approach to eliminate CSCs. The H90, P245, H4C4, GV5, RO5429083 are IgG1 types of monoclonal antibodies (mAbs) directed towards the human CD44 and identified in a constant region of human CD44 receptor [206]. Thus, combining the advanced clinical setting of CSCs targeting mAbs with novel anticancer drugs and conventional cytotoxic drugs shows a very promising strategy to eradicate CSCs, bulk tumour and differentiated progenitors cells in cancer patients [207].

Another stem cell marker CD133 is a transmembrane glycoprotein, which is also known as Prominin-1. CD133$^+$ subpopulations have been shown to be considerably more tumorigenic than CD133$^-$ compartments, which form the bulk tumour in glioblastoma. The marker has also been reported in metastatic colorectal cancer, ovarian cancer and gastric carcinoma (Table **1**). Previous studies suggest that a subpopulation of CD133-positive cancer cells have a significant role in resistance to anticancer drugs [208]. Moreover, radiation-exposed CD133$^+$ hepatic carcinoma cells show enhanced radioresistance compared with CD133$^-$ cells [209]. Polymeric NPs loaded with Curcumin have been shown to significantly reduce the growth of CD133$^+$ CSC population in malignant brain tumours [210]. Moreover, Salinomycin-loaded nanocarriers conjugated with CD133 aptamers (targeting ligand) have been reported to selectively inhibit CD133$^+$ osteosarcoma both *in vitro* and *in vivo* [211]. Previous studies have shown that a high level of ALDH activity is associated with enhanced tumorigenicity and chemoresistance in the CSCs, due to the increased expression and activity of multiple or distinct ALDH isozymes. The increased activity of ALDH1A1 and ALDH3A1 isozymes has been associated with the development of resistance to tumour cell populations. To address this issue, ALDH inhibitors (e.g., 4-Amino-4-Methyl-2-Pentyne-1-AL (AMPAL) and 2-methyl-5-(methylsulfanyl)-5-oxopentan-2-aminium) have been developed which particularly target the ALDH1A1 and ALDH3A1 isozymes, resulting in the inhibition of chemoresistance in the CSCs [212]. It has also been found that ALDHs are preferentially expressed in the CD133[+] subpopulation and could be used to better characterize the tumorigenic CD133[+] CSC population in liver cancers [213 - 215]. Therefore, ALDH can be used as a targeting moiety for delivering drugs to the CSCs and to treat various cancer types. In this regard, nanocarriers play a potential role in directly targeting the ALDH, which is overexpressed in Glioblastoma Multiforme (GBM) cells. Hence, treating GBM with biomaterial containing anti-ALDH may reduce the amount of brain cancer stem cells (BCSCs) through suppressing ALDH activity [216]. Thus, curcumin-loaded chitosan-PLGA NPs modified with sialic acid to permeate the blood-brain barrier and modified with anti-ALDH were designed to target the GBM cells to inhibit the proliferation of glioblastoma cells and BCSCs [217]. Moreover, nanoparticles loaded with drugs like decitabine, a DNA hypermethylation inhibitor and a Hedgehog signalling inhibitor have been developed successfully to target the ALDH to inhibit the CSCs of breast cancer [218, 219]. CD133 can specifically be targeted using CIK cells bound with Bispecific Antibody (BsAb) against CD3/CD133 for successful treatment of cancers. The BsAb is a novel antibody having the ability to target two different antigens and moderate specific killing effects by particularly redirecting effector cells to targeting cells, leading to significant anti-CSCs activity, which is an auspicious way to antitumor immunity with synergistic effects [220, 221].

2.3.2. Targeting Signalling Pathways (Wnt/β-catenin, Notch, TGF-β and Hedgehog Pathways) in CSCs

The cell signalling can be described as a group of molecules in a cell that work together to control all the cellular functions like cell division. When one molecule of a signalling pathway receives a signal, it activates subsequent molecules [222]. The ability of cells to receive and correctly respond to the signals is the basis of development, tissue repair, immunity, as well as cell division. An error in the signalling process can lead to diseases like cancer, autoimmunity and diabetes [223, 224]. By understanding cell-signalling processes and correcting them, the related diseases can be treated.

Signalling by the Wnt family of secreted glycol-lipoproteins is one of the fundamental mechanisms that direct cell proliferation, cell polarity and cell fate determination during embryonic development and tissue homeostasis [225, 226]. When a Wnt ligand binds to the transmembrane complex comprising the Frizzled receptor, the Wnt/β-catenin pathway becomes activated and leads to binding of the low-density lipoprotein-related receptor followed by suppression of glycogen synthase kinase-3β-binding protein, thereby improving the stability of β-catenin, which then accumulates and is translocated to the nucleus. This accumulation of β-catenin in the cell nucleus ultimately leads to the activation of various genes such as c-Myc and cyclin D1 [227]. Deviant activation of the Wnt/β-catenin signalling pathways has been reported in several types of cancers such as ovarian, colon and breast cancer [228]. Therefore, selective targeting of Wnt/β-catenin signalling pathway has been considered as a therapeutic strategy for the treatment of various types of cancers. Curcumin-loaded PLGA nanocarriers have been reported to increase apoptotic effects in Cisplatin-resistant ovarian cancer cells by suppressing Wnt/β-catenin signalling component β-catenin [229]. Reports also showed that 5-Fluorouracil loaded nanocarriers can effectively inhibit the peritoneal dissemination of colorectal cancer cells, which overexpress Wnt/β-catenin signalling components [230, 231].

The Notch signalling pathway is a highly maintained cell signalling system present in most animals. The Notch receptor is a single-pass transmembrane receptor protein and it has four types, viz. NOTCH1, NOTCH2, NOTCH3 and NOTCH4. This pathway controls a broad spectrum of events, such as cell differentiation decisions and the formation of precise tissue patterns [232]. Notch signalling also plays an important role in regulating stem cell maintenance and differentiation [233, 234]. A study shows that the inhibition of Notch signalling sharply decreases self-renewal, clonogenic and the tumorigenic potential of glioblastoma CSCs [235]. Moreover, suppression of Notch signalling leads to a decrease of the CSC-like subpopulation and increases the susceptibility of CSCs to radiation-induced apoptosis in glioblastomas [236]. The Notch signalling can be inhibited by γ-secretase inhibitors, inhibitory peptides and antibodies [237]. Drug conjugated Mesoporous Silica Nanoparticles (MSNPs) have been reported to markedly enhance the cytotoxicity of the drug by selectively targeting the Notch signalling pathways in various cancer cell types, such as cervical and breast cancer cells [238]. Jagged1-*si*RNAs-loaded chitosan nanocarriers have been reported to selectively inhibit ovarian cancer both *in vitro* and *in vivo* by selectively targeting the Notch signalling pathway. Jagged1 has also been called as CD339 and is a cell surface ligand that interacts with a receptor in the highly conserved Notch signalling pathway [239].

TGF-β signalling pathway is involved in many cellular processes like cell growth, cell differentiation, apoptosis and cellular homeostasis. When TGF-β ligands bind to a type-II receptor, they recruit and phosphorylate type I receptor. The type-I receptor then phosphorylates receptor-regulated SMADs (R-SMADs) which can now bind the co-SMAD with SMAD4. R-SMAD/co-SMAD complexes accumulate in the nucleus where they act as transcription factors and participate in the regulation of target gene expression [240]. TGF-β signalling pathway has been reported to be involved in the maintenance and function of CSCs from different types of cancers [241, 242]. Hence, selective targeting of TGF-β signalling pathways may be considered as an effective therapeutic strategy for the treatment of various types of cancer. It has been reported that polyethyleneimine/PEG-conjugated MSNPs loaded with LY364947 (a TGF-β inhibitor) provided significantly improved therapeutic efficiency in tumour xenograft models compared to the treatment with free LY364947 [243]. Moreover, it has also been reported that Gold (Au) Nanoparticles (NPs) i.e., AuNPs have the ability to weaken the immunosuppressive function of TGF-β, resulting in an increased number and frequency of tumour-infiltrating T lymphocytes. These observations indicate that AuNPs can be a promising immune modulator by inhibiting the immunosuppressive function of TGF-β1 signalling pathway [244].

The Hedgehog (Hh) signalling pathway transmits information to embryonic cells required for proper cell differentiation. Different parts of the embryo have different concentrations of Hh signalling proteins. The functional significance of this signalling pathway is proven by an increase in birth defects and malignancies with aberrant activation of this pathway in adults [245, 246]. Humans have three different Hh homologs with different spatial and temporal distribution patterns: Desert Hh (Dhh), Indian Hh (Ihh) and Sonic Hh (Shh) [247]. The Hh signalling is initiated by Hh binding to the 12-transmembrane receptor Patched 1, which frees its forbiddance on Smoothened (Smo), ending in the nuclear localization of DNA-binding Gli transcription factors in target cells [248]. Abrupt activation of the Hh signalling pathway has been reported in various cancer types [249, 250]. Therefore, targeting the Hh signalling pathway may provide an effective therapeutic approach in the treatment of various cancers. A polymeric nanoparticle loaded with Gli antagonist (HPI-1) has been reported to effectively inhibit the growth and invasion of CD133+ cells in liver cancers [251]. Moreover, herbal extract Anthothecol loaded PLGA NPs have been reported to inhibit cell proliferation and colony formation and induce apoptosis in pancreatic CSCs by modulating Hh signalling pathway [252]. These reports show that the Hh signalling targeted nanoparticles might be an effective therapeutic approach in the treatment of cancer.

2.4. Agents Affecting the Microenvironment Signals

The overall surrounding of a tumour including blood vessels, signalling molecules and the extracellular matrix is known as the tumour microenvironment. The microenvironment is always in interaction with the tumour and the tumour can influence the microenvironment by releasing extracellular signals and various other chemicals [253]. CSCs interact with tumour cells by releasing a chemokine i.e., C-X-C chemokine Ligand 12 (CXCL12). The chemokine binding to its receptor i.e., C-X-C chemokine Receptor 4 (CXCR4) and helps in migration, invasion and survival of normal and malignant cells [254]. In human breast cancer, stromal fibroblasts release CXCL12. It helps grow the tumour in two ways: Firstly, it promotes angiogenesis by enrolling endothelial progenitor cells into the tumour mass and secondly, by acting directly on tumour cells through CXCR4 [255]. Moreover, tumour microenvironment is composed of stromal cells (like fibroblasts, mesenchymal stromal cells) and immune cells (like T and B cells, Tumour-associated macrophages) [256]. The immune cells play an essential role in ignited inflammation in the tumour microenvironment. The tumour microenvironment infiltrates by various immune cell types and the active tumour-immune cell interplay effectuates a rich milieu of growth factors and cytokines. Basically, this complicated cross-talk initiates the favourable condition for tumour cell proliferation, metastasis and survival [257]. Additionally, the presence of intra-tumoral T cells is a positive prognostic marker in many cancers, while studies of B cell have been challenging due to the lack of common phenotypic markers, making tumour-specific T cells fabricate the promising live drug therapy for cancer [258, 259]. Although tumours express various types of growth factors that help suppress T-cell activation towards their own cells through aberrant signalling via immune checkpoints including PD-1/PD-L1, T-cell Immunoglobulin and Mucin domain-3 (TIM-3), Cytotoxic T Lymphocyte-associated Antigen-4 (CTLA-4), B7-H3, Lymphocyte Activation Gene-3 (LAG-3) and OX40 are commonly involved with this tumorigenic crosstalk in the tumour microenvironment [260]. However, stromal cells form a substantial component of the microenvironment influencing hypoxia, migration of immune cells and the metastatic behaviour of tumour cells [261]. Therefore, a profound understanding of the multidisciplinary functions of the various immune cell as well as stromal cell types thus confers through developing progressive anticancer therapeutic strategies. Recently, various types of chemotherapeutic agents have been investigated to block the microenvironment signalling including TKIs and mAbs for growth factors, Bortezomib for hypoxic cytokines and Repertaxin for inflammatory cytokines and chemokines signalling [262 - 264].

Understanding the role of CXCL12 and CXCR4 in the functioning of CSCs, researchers have developed agents to block them. Plerixafor, also known as AMD3100 is one of the most widely studied CXCR4 inhibitors and a hematopoietic stem cell mobilizer. Previous studies report that it can induce a rapid mobilization of hematopoietic stem cells and progenitor cells into the blood in mice and humans, curb the growth of intracranial glioblastoma and medulloblastoma xenografts by raising apoptosis and lessening the proliferation of tumour cells and can reduce the intraperitoneal spreading of epithelial ovarian cancer [265 - 267]. CTCE-9908 is a 17 amino acid peptide CXCR4 antagonist that has been shown to block the interaction of the CXCR4 receptor with CXCL12 and has been reported to be effective in reducing both tumour growth and metastasis in inflammatory breast cancer, oesophageal carcinoma and in prostate cancer [268 - 270].

NOX-A12, an RNA oligonucleotide in L-configuration, which is developed by Noxxon Pharma is an anticancer drug that neutralizes CXCL12 by blocking CXCL12 signalling through CXCR4 and CXCR7 receptors [271]. Research has shown that NOX-A12 suppresses CXCL12-induced chemotaxis of chronic lymphocytic leukaemia cells and causes chemosensitization by targeting a key chemokine in the tumour microenvironment leading to block tumour protection and tumour repair mechanism. Moreover, reports suggest that this compound has the potential to improve tumour response in glioblastoma multiform animal model after irradiation [272, 273].

Previous studies have shown that CXCR4 induces an increased expression of Vascular Endothelial Growth Factor (VEGF) in tissues through the activation of PI3K/Akt pathway. As mentioned earlier, the microenvironment promotes tumour angiogenesis, which is essential for CSC survival and tumour growth. Targeting VEGF reduces the vasculature of tumours, decreases tumour growth and disruption of the CSC niche [274]. Bevacizumab, Pazopanib, Sorafenib and Sunitinib are the VEGF inhibitors that FDA has already approved for clinical application. Fruquintinib (HMPL-013), a selective antagonist of the Vascular Endothelial Growth Factor Receptor (VEGFR) family, is currently in Phase II clinical studies [275].

Due to the increased cell division, increased metabolic activity and poor vascular perfusion of tumours, the microenvironment becomes acidic [276]. The literature reports suggest that this acidic microenvironment offers a selective advantage to the cancer cells over the normal tissues and contributes to drug resistance [277, 278]. The acidic pH of the tumours may help in two ways for drug targeting: Firstly, in delivering drugs and drug carriers that have specificity for the acid environment and secondly, by sensitizing the cancer cells to anticancer drugs by changing the pH of the tumour [279]. Tumour tissue in solid cancers usually expresses an acidic pH comparable to non-tumour tissue. Since normal tissue has a pH 7.4, this variation can then be oppressed for initiating drug release in the more acidic tumour tissue [280]. The drug release is mainly achieved by the fusion of an acid-sensitive linker between the carrier and drug, which facilitates drug release at a faintly acidic tumour environment of cancerous cells [281].

Previous studies have proven the efficacy of anticancer drug-loaded nanocarriers responsive to the acidic environment of the tumour, such as liposomes, micelles, polymers and inorganic nanoparticles [282, 283]. Moreover, to enhance the targeting efficiency of drug carriers in tumour microenvironment, the outer layer includes pH-responsive antibodies, cell-penetrating peptides [284, 285]. The H7K(R2)2 has been reported as tumour specific pH-sensitive peptide, acting as a targeting ligand, which could be responding to the acidic pH environment in glioma and possessing cell-penetrating peptide characteristics. This peptide was used to modify pH-sensitive liposomes loaded with Doxorubicin (DOX-PS--H7K(R2)2). The pH-triggered doxorubicin release from the pH-responsive liposomes and targeting effect within acidic conditions has been demonstrated by *in vitro* experiments [286].

Moreover, sodium bicarbonate, a systemic alkalizer has been shown to prevent or slow down the transition from in situ to invasive cancer [287]. The pH of tumour microenvironment also can be raised by administering inhibitors for pH-regulatory pathways like Carbonic anhydrase-IX (CAIX). Phase III clinical trial has suggested that CAIX can also be used for the survival of patients with high-risk non-metastatic renal cell carcinoma [288].

2.5. Modulators of MicroRNAs and their Implication in CSCs Regulation

MicroRNAs or *mi*RNAs are small non-coding RNAs of 20-24 nucleotides in length that stop the transcription process by degrading their target mRNAs and/or inhibiting their translation in the post-transcriptional level. This process has a broad range of effects over self-renewal, differentiation and division of cells [289]. The *mi*RNAs can modify several signalling pathways that have the potential to transform stem cells into CSCs. The *mi*RNAs regulate different properties of CSCs like cell-cycle exit, differentiation, anti-stress mechanisms, EMT, migration and invasion, which increase the tumour initiation and metastatic potential [290]. The differential nature of *mi*RNA makes them probable biomarkers for the cancer prognosis and their selectivity in directing the properties of CSCs makes them attainable targets for therapeutic mediation [291]. Moreover, *mi*RNA could act as potential targets in cancer treatment, thus manipulating *mi*RNAs could be a promising strategy for killing CSCs or repeal of EMT phenotype of cancerous cells. Typically, *mi*RNAs are tightly deregulated in human cancers [292]. The dysregulation of *mi*RNAs in CSCs accidentally exhibits a high level of messenger RNA (mRNA), which is specific to oncogene or tumour suppressor genes [293]. Targeting the oncogenic *mi*RNAs can be acquired by inhibition of antisense oligonucleotide [294]. Recent evidence illustrates that the appearance of *mi*R-21 is markedly upward and *mi*R-145 is downward in many CSCs. Therefore, knockdown of *mi*R-21 and *mi*R-145 inhibits cell proliferation, migration and tumour growth of many cancers including colon, lung, breast, ovarian cancer [295 - 298]. Simultaneously, *mi*R-21 and *mi*R-145 modulate the chemosensitivity of anticancer drugs Sunitinib and Demethoxycurcumin [299, 300].

For the tumour suppressor gene p53, *mi*R-34 is a target. But, in many cancers, the *mi*R-34 becomes down-regulated and the p53 gene becomes less effective and it fails to control the cancer growth [301]. Studies have shown that increasing the expression of *mi*R-34a inhibits the clonogenic expansion, tumour regeneration and metastasis in CD44[+] prostate cancer cells. Moreover, reports also suggest that transfection of synthetic *mi*R-34a inhibited clonogenic expansion and tumour regeneration in CD44[+] non-small cell lung cancer cell lines, *in vivo* [302, 303]. Thus, *mi*RNA based therapy that can correct abnormal transcriptions at CSCs level, shows great potential for cancer cure.

2.6. Apoptotic Inducers of CSCs

Apoptosis is the process of programmed cell death that occurs as a normal and controlled part of an organism's growth or development [304]. Apoptosis takes place through a complex signalling mechanism and is dedicatedly balanced or regulated in a physiological context [305]. The failure of this regulation often leads to the initiation or progression of pathological disorders like autoimmune diseases, neurodegeneration or cancer [306].

Induction of apoptosis in CSCs can be activated by two pathways i.e., extrinsic pathway and intrinsic pathway hold great promises for cancer therapy. Therefore, researchers have developed many compounds to target intrinsic and extrinsic apoptotic pathways [307, 308]. The extrinsic pathway is activated through the binding of extracellular proapoptotic ligands to cell surface receptors, known as death receptors like TNF (Tumour Necrosis Factor)-Related Apoptosis-Inducing Ligand (TRAIL) receptors, CD95 and Nerve Growth Factor Receptor (NGFR), while the intrinsic pathway is induced by a sort of stress signals that provoke the DNA and cellular damage, like ionizing radiation, cytotoxic agents and growth factor withdrawal [309 - 311]. Activation of the death receptor CD95 using trimeric human TRAIL leads to Caspase-8, a cysteine proteases enzyme activation [312]. Once activated, the enzyme either directly cleaves and activates effector caspase-3 (death protease) or alternatively processes Bid (i.e., an abundant pro-apoptotic protein of the B-cell lymphoma 2 (Bcl-2) family that is crucial for death receptor-mediated apoptosis in many cell systems) into the active fragment tBid, which translocate to mitochondrial membranes to initiate mitochondrial outer membrane permeabilization [313, 314]. Co-administration of TRAIL with various anticancer agents has been reported to effectively remove CSCs. Therefore, the combination of recombinant TRAIL together with cytotoxic principles such as cisplatin and bortezomib has been shown to enhance the apoptosis of CSCs [315 - 317].

NF-κB is a transcription factor linked to the control of apoptosis signalling known to inhibit cell apoptosis and promote cell proliferation, tumour promotion, angiogenesis and metastasis [318, 319]. It has been reported that with the inhibition of NF-κB with agents like parthenolide, pyrrolidine-dithiocarbamate and its analogue Diethyl-dithiocarbamate in breast cancer, preferentially the CSCs are eliminated [320]. Moreover, co-administration of the proteasome inhibitor MG-132 with Idarubicin induces apoptosis preferentially in the leukemic stem cells population [321]. Increasing recognition of apoptotic signal effector pathways in CSCs paves the way for the development of more specific inducers targeting key signalling components. Currently, a wide range of specific CSC-targeting agents including natural compounds (Genistein), synthetic compounds (Aspirin and IMD-0354), antibiotics (Salinomycin), antibodies (Bevacizumab) and Oligonucleotides (AS-ODN) have been explored [322]. Thus, combined applications of these agents targeting CSC apoptosis are an important advantage of improving their antitumor efficacy.

3. CHALLENGES OF DEVELOPING THE ABOVE STRATEGIES

The discovery of CSCs in human cancer threatened our current understanding of cancer reoccurrence, metastasis and drug resistance [323, 324]. Resistance to therapy along with cancer relapse and metastasis comprises some of the major clinical challenges attributed to a subpopulation of CSCs for successful cancer treatment [325]. Conventional cancer therapy can target only the bulk of the sensitive cancer cells, which are in the rapidly dividing phase. These therapeutic strategies induce apoptosis or death of many cancer cells, whereas CSCs survive by remaining in the G0 phase and give rise to the second-line tumour with a higher risk of drug resistance [326]. The mechanisms by which CSCs outbreak anticancer therapies include the removal of chemotherapeutic agents by drug-efflux pumps, upgraded repair function of DNA damage, stimulation of mitogenic/anti-apoptotic pathways, evasion of immune response, cellular plasticity, the adaptation to a hostile microenvironment as well as the main features of CSCs like stemness and EMT [327, 328]. Recently, CSC has gained much attention due to the recognition of key molecules responsible for controlling the distinctive properties of CSC populations [329]. The development of novel strategies to target CSCs populations is in demand for the therapeutic termination of CSCs and the full eradication of cancers [330]. However, proper identification of CSCs from cancer cells is a serious problem in the field of novel technologies. In order to design or develop an effective therapeutic intervention for complete eradication of cancers, it is very crucial to have the effective strategies to identify CSCs from the bulk population of cancer cells [331].

Moreover, in order to design or develop an effective therapeutics; it is very urgent for understanding the biology of CSCs especially the signalling pathways that are involved in their self-renewal mechanisms [332]. Like normal stem cells, CSCs exhibit significant phenotypic homogeneity and functional heterogeneity and that CSCs progeny can show diverse cellular plasticity [333]. The cancer cell heterogeneity and high plasticity intensify the objection of suitable targeting moieties for many cancers by not only CSCs but also many non-CSC cells [334]. Such non-CSCs are spontaneously de-differentiated into CSCs by a phenomenon known as cancer cell plasticity [335]. Also, the identification of possible target sites of CSCs is difficult due to the lack of actual specific markers, cancer cell plasticity, cell signalling pathways and DNA repair mechanisms making the targeting CSCs to eradicate cancers challenging [336, 337]. Therefore, challenges associated with novel therapeutics for targeting CSCs are discussed below:

The existence of CSCs and their association with chemo resistance as well as relapse has led to a search for active drug molecules to eliminate these cells [338]. The discovery and development of targeted new chemical entities and new biological entities against CSCs remain challenging, although few molecules have completed Phase II human clinical trials and have been shifted to Phase III trials to determine the efficacy and safety of these new drug molecules [339]. However, the new drug molecules pose several pitfalls including low aqueous solubility, stability and nonspecific toxicity; which limit their applications in cancer therapy. To overcome the known shortcomings of new anticancer drug molecules, the term nanomedicine has gained much attraction [340]. Nanomedicines provide fundamental benefits over current small-molecule pharmaceuticals employed in clinical trials such as enhanced bioavailability, extended half-life of the drug as well as minimized non-specific toxicities [341]. Moreover, nanomedicines can encapsulate the high concentration of chemotherapeutic agents and deliver them within the cancer cells including CSCs appropriately overcoming drug resistance functionalities of CSCs [342]. Currently, CSCs target specificity, cellular internalization, and macrophage uptake are the major problems associated with the nanomedicines [343, 344]. Thus, the surface modified nanomedicines (surface modified with specific targeting moiety like ligand, antibodies or hydrophilic segment) may increase the target specificity as well as cellular internalization by binding with the overexpressed receptor, increase cell-specific uptake and deliver sufficient amount of drug to target cells [345 - 347].

It is well known that CSCs express different surface markers that can be used for their identification and to provide therapeutic targets for the development of specific cytotoxic molecules [348]. CSCs can often be identified by several cell surface markers such as CD44, CD47, CD123, CD326 (epithelial cell adhesion molecule), CD133 [349, 350]. However, in most of the cases, these markers are also expressed by healthy adult stem cells that make it hard to differentiate and target CSC only which pose major challenges to eradicate CSCs [351]. Currently, multiparametric flow cytometry is the most common method used to identify CSCs from normal stem cells underlying the expression of specific markers or functional properties by Fluorescence-Activated Cell Sorting (FACS) [352, 353]. Notably, several molecular signalling pathways that govern normal cell haemostasis are highly regulated, but surprisingly many of these pathways are abnormally activated or become dysfunctional in CSCs [354]. It has been speculated that signalling pathways of the stem cell i.e., Wnt/β-catenin, Notch, Hh and TGFβ/BMP play a prominent role in the CSCs homeostasis and critically regulate the self-renewal or survival of CSCs [355]. These cell signalling pathways often exhibit significant crosstalk during embryogenesis, which is the major issue in the development of new agents that targeting the CSCs signalling pathways [356]. For example, in the experiment of glioblastoma cells along with patient specimens, the inhibition of Notch signalling resulted in the down regulation of its target gene Hes1, which upregulated the GLI transcription in the Hh pathway [357]. Thus, preventing the crosstalk among the cell signalling pathways can modulate better therapeutic targeting against CSCs.

The tumour microenvironment plays a significant role in regulating the signalling cascade of CSC phenotype during progression and differentiation of CSCs [358]. The microenvironment is mainly composed of the extracellular matrix and tightly regulates the CSCs, leading to create a CSC niche [359]. In the CSC niche, several microenvironment components can communicate with CSCs, holding their self-renewal capacity and promoting drug resistance [360]. The key signalling molecules i.e., growth factors such as VEGF, Epidermal Growth Factor (EGF), and Fibroblast Growth Factors (FGF) promote tumour angiogenesis and induce peripheral immune tolerance. The hypoxic cytokines include Hypoxia-Inducible Factor-1α (HIF-1α), which mediate multiple biological effects of hypoxia in tissues. The inflammatory cytokine and chemokines such as IL-1β, IL-6, IL-8 and IL-17 activate the NF-κB/STAT3 pathways in tumour and stromal cells to prompt the CSCs microenvironmental signal that decreases overall survival and increase the drug resistance in cancer suffering patients [361 - 363]. The IL-6 frequently interacts with CSCs and maintains the stemness of CSCs [364]. Similarly, by NFκB/STAT3 pathways, IL-17-IL-17R interaction in Glioma Stem Cells (GSCs) induces an autocrine and/or paracrine cytokine feedback loop that may provide an important signalling pathway for the stemness of GSCs [365]. During the evaluation of these signalling pathways, the crosstalk between the CSCs and microenvironment is critical for tumour progression leading to provide challenges of chemotherapeutic agents to sufficiently prevent the progression, cell invasion and metastasis of CSCs [366]. Thus, crosstalk functionality can turn into a major difficulty in the cancer treatment, as the blocking of one cancer-suited signalling pathway can result in the activation of a secondary survival pathway, which can interfere with the efficacy of an anticancer drug therapy [367].

The CSC chemo resistance mainly occurs due to protection imparted by a high expression of the ABC drug transporters [368]. These multidrug transporters use their drug-efflux functions to toss out the various distinct and structurally unrelated drug molecules at the cost of ATP hydrolysis, lower the intracellular drug concentration and thus being inattentive to the cancer therapy [369]. Normal adult stem cells and CSCs appear to express elevated levels of ABC transporters, thereby excessive levels of ABC transporters allow CSCs to maintain resistance against the current anticancer therapies [370, 371]. The well-known ABC superfamily includes P-gp/ABCB1, MRP/ABCC1 and BCRP/ABCG2 and these are overexpressed in various cancers and are able to efflux a wide range of chemotherapeutic agents leading to drug resistance [372, 373]. The most challenging investigation of altering the multi-drug resistance of CSCs is the inhibition of particular ABC drug transporters [374]. There are three generations of ABCB1 inhibitors that have been designed. All of them proved to be a failure and none of them had any additional effect on prognosis [375]. The several complications might have limited the clinical success of ABC transporter inhibitors including pharmacokinetics alteration and decreased systemic clearance of the anticancer drug as well as side population cells that have a huge potentiality for effluxing Hoechst dye [376, 377]. Moreover, functional redundancy and frequent overexpression of numerous ABC transporter genes like P-gp gene expression can inhibit the function ABC transporter [378].

Currently, *mi*RNAs provide a new avenue in understanding the regulatory mechanisms in CSCs and also play the critical roles in normal stem cell functions during their development [379]. Aberrant expression of *mi*RNAs and their intimation in CSCs exponentially control the key characteristics of CSCs [380, 381]. In addition, *mi*RNA also regulates the function of EMT of CSCs [382]. EMT allows tumour cells to enter the metastatic cascade by altering their molecular and morphological characteristics and it exhibits a wide spectrum that cancer cells keep transiting. Moreover, EMT-borrowed tumour cells promote stem cell properties and display distinct therapeutic resistance. Thus, finding possible *mi*RNA targets for blocking EMT is a prominent challenge for *mi*RNA based therapy [383 - 385]. The efficacy of this therapy is significantly lowered by the unsuitable size of the *mi*RNA gene expression or vector. Thus, it is recommended to improve this technique based on the insertion of synthetic *mi*RNA mimics or optimizing *mi*RNA expression cassettes in diverse virus vectors [386 - 388]. Furthermore, the major obstacles in the development or design of *mi*RNAs based therapies include low bioavailability, limited tissue permeability and payload instability. These pose a major challenge for *in vivo* delivery as well as the fractional reciprocity of *mi*RNAs to their target genes along with the various forms of seed mismatch-pairing. It represents one of the prime challenges in the recognition of *mi*RNA target in both normal and cancerous stem cells [389].

Apoptosis is a genetically controlled mechanism that mediates the equilibrium between cell survival as well as cell death in metazoan by the removal of redundant and unwanted cells [390]. Generally, the apoptotic mechanisms are damaged during cancer development and progression. It is the reason for cancer cells resistance to therapy [391]. Apoptosis can be induced by extrinsic and intrinsic pathways. These pathways are typically deregulated in CSCs and these cells play crucial roles in tumour initiation, progression, cell death resistance, resistance to therapy and tumour recurrence [392]. The better identification of signalling effectors of apoptosis pathways in CSCs overlaid the route for the development or design of more selective inducers targeting components [393]. Multiple compounds have shown anti-CSC ability by activating apoptosis while non-specific targeting, poor efficiency and toxicity issue comprise major challenges leading to deactivate the apoptosis, which is likely responsible for the survival of CSCs [394, 395]. Therefore, exploiting the above apoptotic machinery could be promising strategies for eradicating CSCs tumorigenicity or metastasis, which displays great potentials in cancer therapy.

4. RECENT PATENTS ISSUED IN THE AREA OF CSCS TARGETING

Emerging evidence has suggested that CSCs are the main driver of tumorigenesis and are poised to transform the whole perspective of cancer therapy in the 21st century [396]. The current practice is to eradicate CSCs along with tumour bulk either by monotherapy or combination chemotherapy leading to improve patient survival rate [397]. Consequently, the concept of proper CSCs targeting, hence aspiring to novel strategies in cancer therapeutics, is obtaining significant attraction in the field of cancer research [398]. A profound search for more precise recognition of CSCs along with more effective drug search granted many interesting research patents during the last few years [399]. Accompanying the advances in CSCs research, some patents have been awarded with respect to novel CSC markers, gene expression system, methods to isolate and modulate the CSCs as well as new compounds directly targeting CSCs [400]. Benitah *et al.,* filed a patent on targeting metastasis stem cells by a fatty acid receptor. They identified anticancer agents, particularly for Oral Squamous Cell Cancer (OSCC) metastasis. More particularly, the present invention reveals the use of antibodies or other inhibitors of CD36 expression for the effective treatment against OSCC metastasis and cancer [401]. Hoque *et al.,* filed a patent on methods for treating cancer based on the recognition of pharmaceutical agents that target CSCs. These methods include an efficient amount of a COX2 inhibitor (celecoxib) and an efficient amount of YAP1 inhibitor (verteporfin), which enhance chemotherapeutic responses in cancer patients [402]. Jabbari filed a patent on systems and methods for targeting specific cancer cell subpopulations present in tumour tissue. The system consists of a first component specifically targeting cancer stem cells and a second component for specifically targeting differentiated cancer cells. The first component (free drug) is conjugated to small nanoparticles and the second component (free drug) is encapsulated in the nanoparticles, which can be preferentially taken up by the CSCs without triggering the efflux pump [403]. Shi *et al.,* filed a patent on strategy for targeting glioblastoma stem cells through the TLX-TET3 Axis for a novel therapy of brain cancer. They provided methods or compositions capable of modulating the activity of TLX (NR2E1) by downregulating TLX expression and/or modulating its downstream component Ten Eleven Translocation 3 (TET3) [404]. Kosai *et al.,* filed a patent on targeting CSCs using a viral vector. They suggested that the adenoviral vector comprising CSC-specific promoter can be used for treatment and diagnosis. Furthermore, the present invention provides the methods for recognizing CSCs and provides a labelling agent and a toxic agent for CSCs, containing the adenoviral vector as the active ingredient [405]. Magnani filed a patent on targeting CSC by antibodies. He found antibodies such as HECA-452 and CSC-specific cell surface carbohydrates that bind to E-selectin to contain carbohydrate epitopes i.e., sialyl Lea/x are overexpressed by E-selectin-binding cancers. Such cancers can be treated with antagonists of E-selectin and with immunotherapies that target the sialyl Lea/x domains to block the binding of E-selectin [406]. Yang *et al.,* filed a patent on a new composition in the form of nanoparticles for targeting CSCs. The nanoparticle composition of the present invention comprises a central core containing magnetic iron oxide (Fe_3O_4) nanoparticles, shell portion containing chemotherapeutic agent and the surface of the said shell modified with the antibodies capable of binding with a receptor on the cell surface of the target CSCs. Results supported that a combination specificity of the nanoparticle composition synergistically inhibits the CSCs [407]. Utku *et al.,* filed a patent on targeting CSCs by the use of etoposide and prodrugs thereof. The present invention pertains to the use of podophyllotoxin derivatives, such as CAP7.1 for inhibition or prevention of the growth and survival of CSCs. Moreover, the analogue of etoposide called CAP7.1, which is suitable for treating drug-resistant (etoposide resistant) tumour, is able to reduce drug resistance, particularly multidrug resistance [408]. Xing *et al.,* filed a patent on the use of omeprazole for the preparation of CSC inhibitors. They designed a technical scheme where CD133 is used as a molecular marker to obtain LCSCs (liver cancer stem cells) and at the same time, the experimental animal tumour model was constructed to inspect the inhibitory effects of omeprazole. Results revealed that by the application of omeprazole, the proliferation of the LCSC cells could be directly inhibited [409]. Li *et al.,* filed a patent on discovering new compounds and compositions for directly targeting CSCs. They found that preparation of furan and naphthalene compounds (particulate form), pure polymorphs and pharmaceutical compositions could selectively inhibit the CSCs and STAT3 pathways and are useful for treatment or prevention of reoccurrence of cancer [410]. Udugamasooriya *et al.,* filed a patent on new pharmaceutical compositions and methods specifically targeting CSCs. They found pharmaceutical compositions containing peptoids of general formula (I), (II), or (III) capable of reducing the proliferation of CSCs and method of detecting and treating cancerous cell masses by the use of peptoids [411]. Cheresh *et al.,* filed a patent on discovering new compositions and methods for targeting and killing ALPHA-V BETA-3-positive CSCs and treatment of drug-resistant cancers. They found targeting cell surface-expressed ALPHAV BETA-3 polypeptides in CSCs as a very promising way to treat cancers. In this regard, they used an antibody (also comprises an Fc portion) that can specifically bind to human ALPHA-V BETA-3 and control antibody-dependent cell-mediated cytotoxicity [412]. Li *et al.,* filed a patent on developing a novel class of STAT3 pathway inhibitors to selectively target CSCs. They found that naphtho[2,3-b]furan-4,9-dione and related compounds can directly inhibit the STAT3 pathway leading to target CSCs and treat malignant diseases [413]. Yun *et al.,* filed a patent on targeting CSC and cancer cell by the use of the gene expression system. They found the gene expression system to be specifically expressed in CSCs as well as cancer cells and developed recombinant adenovirus, which specifically kills the CSCs and cancer cells using the gene expression system [414]. The applicable patents on the regulation of CSCs and cancer therapy by CSCs are represented in Table **3**.

Table 3. Recent Patents Issued in the Area of CSCs Targeting.

Inventors	Title	Patent Number	Ref (s)
Benitah, S.A., Angulo, G.P., Martin, A.C., Martin, M.P.	Targeting metastasis stem cells through a fatty acid receptor (CD36)	US20190106503	[401]
Hoque, M.O., Sidransky, D., Oki, A.	Pharmaceutical agents targeting cancer stem cells	US20190091202	[402]
Jabbari, E.	Drug delivery system and method for targeting cancer stem cells	US20190054034	[403]

(Table 3) contd.....

Inventors	Title	Patent Number	Ref (s)
Shi, Y., Cui, Q., Yang, S.	Targeting glioblastoma stem cells through the TLX-TET3 Axis	US20190032055	[404]
Kosai, K., Wang, Y.	Viral vector targeting cancer stem cells	US20180346929	[405]
Magnani, J.L.	Antibodies for targeting cancer stem cells and treating aggressive cancers	US20180318325	[406]
Yang, M., Liu, D.	Nanoparticle composition for use in targeting cancer stem cells and method for treatment of cancer	US20180193485	[407]
Utku, N., Gullans, S.R.	Etoposide and prodrugs thereof for use in targeting cancer stem cells	US20180042952	[408]
Xing, J., Jiang, Z.	Application of omeprazole in preparation of liver cancer stem cell inhibitor	CN108685919	[409]
Li, J.C., David, L., Li, Y., Li, W.	New compound and composition for targeting cancer stem cell	CN107721958	[410]
Udugamasooriya, G.D., Raymond, A., Minna, J.	Compositions and methods of targeting cancer stem cells	WO2018053472	[411]
Cheresh, D., Wettersten, H.	Compositions and methods for targeting and killing ALPHA-V BETA-3-positive cancer stem cells (CSCs) and treating drug-resistant cancers	WO2018183894	[412]
Li, J.C., Jiang, Z., Harry, R., Li, Y., Liu, J., Li, W.	Novel group of STAT3 pathway inhibitors and cancer stem cell pathway inhibitors	JP2018076349	[413]
Yun, O.C., Oh, J.E.	Gene expression system for targeting cancer stem cell and cancer cell	KR20180044141	[414]

CURRENT & FUTURE DEVELOPMENTS

Researchers are utilizing their time and resources for the identification of CSCs of various cancers and finding ways to eliminate them without damaging the healthy cells. In this aspect, they have achieved success to some extent as a few therapeutic agents are in clinical trials and are supposed to go for mass production very soon. However, we still do not have a rugged system to attain both of the goals. Hence, the researchers are looking for newer techniques to identify CSCs and drug molecules to eliminate them effectively with lower costs to bear. Thus, more specific targeting therapies that can particularly target CSCs but spare normal stem cells are urgently needed. Some newer techniques such as the cellular DNA barcoding technology is helping researchers to better understand how tumour cells respond to therapy by knowing the complexity of tumour heterogeneity and gaining insights into temporal tumour evolution. The Clustered Regularly Interspaced Short Palindromic Repeats and CRISPR-associated (CRISPR-Cas) technology are also helping the researchers in generating large libraries of targeting constructs by genomic editing systems to discover novel therapeutic targets in cancer using Loss-of-Function (LoF) and Gain-of-Function (GoF) screens, which drastically reduce the time and cost required to design a new drug molecule for CSC targeted therapy. Also, the immunotherapy has become one of the most promising targeted therapeutic strategies for eliminating CSCs that utilizes many aspects of the immune system. The latest technique involves the creation and/or modification of antibodies for CSC specificity due to their innate ability to target very specific, CSC-associated antigens. The CSC targeted immunotherapies include the use of monoclonal Antibodies (mAbs), Bi-specific monoclonal Antibodies (BsAbs), Bi-specific T-cell Engagers (BiTEs), and Chimeric Antigen Receptors (CARs). In addition, clarifying the considerable crosstalk between cell signalling pathways and microenvironment, inherent plasticity or heterogeneity and hypoxia are critical for designing effective or novel therapeutic approaches. Therefore, future developments should be focused on the combination therapies i.e., combinations of drugs that target CSCs together with chemo/radiotherapy or immunotherapy or molecular targeted therapy or microenvironment modulating agents that affect the multiple pathways of tumour and represent more promising strategies to control cancer progression. We hope the application of these newer technologies will definitely help researchers to develop a complete system for the identification of CSCs and ways to eliminate or control CSCs overpopulation to cure cancer soon.

LIST OF ABBREVIATIONS

SCs	Stem Cells
CSCs	Cancer Stems Cells
DDR	DNA Damage Response
TGF	Transforming Growth Factor
BMP	Bone Morphogenetic Proteins
EGFR	Epidermal Growth Factor Receptor
MAPK	Mitogen-Activated Protein Kinase
NF-κB	Nuclear Factor kappa activated B
STAT3	Signal Transducer and Activator of Transcription 3
EMT	Epithelial-Mesenchymal Transition
miRNA	MicroRNA
AML	Acute Myeloid Leukaemia
P13K	Phosphatidylinositol 3-Kinase
mTOR	mammalian Target Of Rapamycin
ABC	ATP-Binding Cassette
P-gp	P-glycoprotein

TKIs	Tyrosine Kinase Inhibitors
siRNA	Small Interfering RNA
EGCG	Epigallocatechin-3-Gallate
BCRP	Breast Cancer Resistance Protein
MRP	Multidrug Resistance Protein
IPT	Insulin Potentiated Therapy
IGF	Insulin-like Growth Factor
TKRs	Tyrosine Kinase Receptors
IRs	Insulin Receptors
NPs	Nanoparticles
CIK	Cytokine-Induced Killer
NK	Natural Killer
DCs	Dendritic Cells
γδT	Gamma Delta T
CTLs	Cytotoxic T Lymphocytes
IL	Interleukin
IFN-γ	Interferon-Gamma
PD-1	Programmed Cell Death-1
PD-L1	Programmed Cell Death-Ligand 1
ALDH	Aldehyde Dehydrogenase
MHC	Major Histocompatibility Complex
CD	Cluster of Differentiation
mAbs	monoclonal Antibodies
AMPAL	4-Amino-4-Methyl-2-Pentyne-1-AL
GBM	Glioblastoma Multiforme
BCSCs	Brain Cancer Stem Cells
HPI	Hedgehog Signalling Inhibitor
BsAb	Bispecific Antibody
MSNPs	Mesoporous Silica Nanoparticles
AuNPs	Gold Nanoparticles
Hh	Hedgehog
CXCL12	C-X-C chemokine Ligand 12
CXCR4	C-X-C chemokine Receptor 4
TIM-3	T-cell Immunoglobulin and Mucin domain-3
CTLA-4	Cytotoxic T Lymphocyte-Associated Antigen-4

LAG-3	Lymphocyte Activation Gene-3
VEGF	Vascular Endothelial Growth Factor
VEGFR	Vascular Endothelial Growth Factor Receptor
CAIX	Carbonic Anhydrase-IX
mRNA	messenger RNA
TNF	Tumour Necrosis Factor
TRAIL	TNF-Related Apoptosis-Inducing Ligand
NGFR	Nerve Growth Factor Receptor
Bcl-2	B-Cell Lymphoma-2
FACS	Fluorescence-Activated Cell Sorting
EGF	Epidermal Growth Factor
FGF	Fibroblast Growth Factor
GSCs	Glioma Stems Cells
OSCC	Oral Squamous Cell Cancer
TET3	Ten Eleven Translocation 3
LoF	Loss-of-Function
GoF	Gain-of-Function
BiTEs	Bi-specific T-Cell Engagers
CARs	Chimeric Antigen Receptors
CRISPR-Cas	Clustered Regularly Interspaced Short Palindromic Repeats and CRISPR-Associated

CONSENT FOR PUBLICATION

All the authors have equally contributed and given consent to publish this chapter.

FUNDING

This work is financially supported by Dibrugarh University (DU) under the DU Research Fellowship Scheme.

CONFLICT OF INTEREST

Authors declare that there is no conflict of interest. All tables and figures are self-made and original.

ACKNOWLEDGEMENTS

Authors gratefully acknowledge the Dibrugarh University Research Fellowship (DURF) to Sanjoy Das to carry out the research and preparation of this chapter.

REFERENCES

[1]   Chagastelles PC, Nardi NB. Biology of stem cells: An overview. Kidney Int Suppl (2011) 2011; 1(3): 63-7.
[http://dx.doi.org/10.1038/kisup.2011.15] [PMID: 25028627]

[2]   Sada A, Tumbar T. New insights into mechanisms of stem cell daughter fate determination in regenerative tissues. Int Rev Cell Mol Biol 2013; 300: 1-50.
[http://dx.doi.org/10.1016/B978-0-12-405210-9.00001-1] [PMID: 23273858]

[3]   Dang HT, Budhu A, Wang XW. The origin of cancer stem cells. J Hepatol 2014; 60(6): 1304-5.
[http://dx.doi.org/10.1016/j.jhep.2014.03.001] [PMID: 24631602]

[4]   Wicha MS, Liu S, Dontu G. Cancer stem cells: An old idea--a paradigm shift. Cancer Res 2006; 66(4): 1883-90.
[http://dx.doi.org/10.1158/0008-5472.CAN-05-3153] [PMID: 16488983]

[5]   Shiozawa Y, Nie B, Pienta KJ, Morgan TM, Taichman RS. Cancer stem cells and their role in metastasis. Pharmacol Ther 2013; 138(2): 285-93.
[http://dx.doi.org/10.1016/j.pharmthera.2013.01.014] [PMID: 23384596]

[6]   Rycaj K, Tang DG. Cell-of-origin of cancer versus cancer stem cells: Assays and interpretations. Cancer Res 2015; 75(19): 4003-11.
[http://dx.doi.org/10.1158/0008-5472.CAN-15-0798] [PMID: 26292361]

[7]   Li L, Neaves WB. Normal stem cells and cancer stem cells: The niche matters. Cancer Res 2006; 66(9): 4553-7.
[http://dx.doi.org/10.1158/0008-5472.CAN-05-3986] [PMID: 16651403]

[8]   Mayol JF, Loeuillet C, Hérodin F, Wion D. Characterisation of normal and cancer stem cells: One experimental paradigm for two kinds of stem cells. BioEssays 2009; 31(9): 993-1001.
[http://dx.doi.org/10.1002/bies.200900041] [PMID: 19644922]

[9]   Zhang B, Hsu YC. Emerging roles of transit-amplifying cells in tissue regeneration and cancer. Wiley Interdiscip Rev Dev Biol 2017; 6(5): 1-14.
[http://dx.doi.org/10.1002/wdev.282] [PMID: 28670819]

[10] Patel P, Chen EI. Cancer stem cells, tumor dormancy, and metastasis. Front Endocrinol (Lausanne) 2012; 3(125): 125.
[http://dx.doi.org/10.3389/fendo.2012.00125] [PMID: 23109929]

[11] Chang JC. Cancer stem cells: Role in tumor growth, recurrence, metastasis, and treatment resistance. Medicine (Baltimore) 2016; 95(1)(1 Suppl. 1): S20-5.
[http://dx.doi.org/10.1097/MD.0000000000004766] [PMID: 27611935]

[12] Bao B, Ahmad A, Azmi AS, Ali S, Sarkar FH. Overview of cancer stem cells (CSCs) and mechanisms of their regulation: Implications for cancer therapy. Curr Protoc Pharmacol 2013; 61(1): 14.25.1-14.25.14.
[http://dx.doi.org/10.1002/0471141755.ph1425s61] [PMID: 23744710]

[13] Ghiaur G, Gerber J, Jones RJ. Concise review: Cancer stem cells and minimal residual disease. Stem Cells 2012; 30(1): 89-93.
[http://dx.doi.org/10.1002/stem.769] [PMID: 22045578]

[14] Sell S. History of cancer stem cells.Regulatory Networks in Stem Cells Stem Cell Biology and Regenerative Medicine in Regulatory Networks in Stem Cells. 1st ed. Totowa, New Jersey: Humana Press 2009; pp. 495-503.
[http://dx.doi.org/10.1007/978-1-60327-227-8_37]

[15] Sell S. Alpha-fetoprotein, stem cells and cancer: How study of the production of alpha-fetoprotein during chemical hepatocarcinogenesis led to reaffirmation of the stem cell theory of cancer. Tumour Biol 2008; 29(3): 161-80.
[http://dx.doi.org/10.1159/000143402] [PMID: 18612221]

[16]   Sell S. Stem Cells and Cancer: An Introduction. Stem Cells and Cancer. 1ˢᵗ ed. New York: Springer 2009; pp. 1-31.
[http://dx.doi.org/10.1007/978-0-387-89611-3_1]

[17]   Fulawka L, Donizy P, Halon A. Cancer stem cells--the current status of an old concept: Literature review and clinical approaches. Biol Res 2014; 47(1): 66-74.
[http://dx.doi.org/10.1186/0717-6287-47-66] [PMID: 25723910]

[18]   Takebe N, Ivy SP. Controversies in cancer stem cells: Targeting embryonic signaling pathways. Clin Cancer Res 2010; 16(12): 3106-12.
[http://dx.doi.org/10.1158/1078-0432.CCR-09-2934] [PMID: 20530695]

[19]   Xie X, Teknos TN, Pan Q. Are all cancer stem cells created equal? Stem Cells Transl Med 2014; 3(10): 1111-5.
[http://dx.doi.org/10.5966/sctm.2014-0085] [PMID: 25122687]

[20]   Sell S. On the stem cell origin of cancer. Am J Pathol 2010; 176(6): 2584-494.
[http://dx.doi.org/10.2353/ajpath.2010.091064] [PMID: 20431026]

[21]   González-Moles MA, Scully C, Ruiz-Ávila I, Plaza-Campillo JJ. The cancer stem cell hypothesis applied to oral carcinoma. Oral Oncol 2013; 49(8): 738-46.
[http://dx.doi.org/10.1016/j.oraloncology.2013.04.002] [PMID: 23642758]

[22]   Ciurea ME, Georgescu AM, Purcaru SO, *et al.* Cancer stem cells: Biological functions and therapeutically targeting. Int J Mol Sci 2014; 15(5): 8169-85.
[http://dx.doi.org/10.3390/ijms15058169] [PMID: 24821540]

[23]   Rich JN. Cancer stem cells: Understanding tumor hierarchy and heterogeneity. Medicine (Baltimore) 2016; 95(1)(Suppl. 1): S2-7.
[http://dx.doi.org/10.1097/MD.0000000000004764] [PMID: 27611934]

[24]   Hinohara K, Polyak K. Intratumoral heterogeneity: More than just mutations. Trends Cell Biol 2019; 29(7): 569-79.
[http://dx.doi.org/10.1016/j.tcb.2019.03.003] [PMID: 30987806]

[25]   Deshpande N, Rangarajan A. Cancer stem cells: Formidable allies of cancer. Indian J Surg Oncol 2015; 6(4): 400-14.
[http://dx.doi.org/10.1007/s13193-015-0451-7] [PMID: 27081258]

[26]   Ayob AZ, Ramasamy TS. Cancer stem cells as key drivers of tumour progression. J Biomed Sci 2018; 25(1): 20-37.
[http://dx.doi.org/10.1186/s12929-018-0426-4] [PMID: 29506506]

[27]   Alguacil-Núñez C, Ferrer-Ortiz I, García-Verdú E, López-Pirez P, Llorente-Cortijo IM, Sainz B Jr. Current perspectives on the crosstalk between lung cancer stem cells and cancer-associated fibroblasts. Crit Rev Oncol Hematol 2018; 125: 102-10.
[http://dx.doi.org/10.1016/j.critrevonc.2018.02.015] [PMID: 29650269]

[28]   De Francesco EM, Sotgia F, Lisanti MP. Cancer Stem Cells (CSCs): Metabolic strategies for their identification and eradication. Biochem J 2018; 475(9): 1611-34.
[http://dx.doi.org/10.1042/BCJ20170164] [PMID: 29743249]

[29]   Shibata M, Shen MM. The roots of cancer: Stem cells and the basis for tumor heterogeneity. Bioessays 2013; 35(3): 253-60.
[http://dx.doi.org/10.1002/bies.201200101] [PMID: 23027425]

[30]   Shackleton M, Quintana E, Fearon ER, Morrison SJ. Heterogeneity in cancer: Cancer stem cells versus clonal evolution. Cell 2009; 138(5): 822-9.
[http://dx.doi.org/10.1016/j.cell.2009.08.017] [PMID: 19737509]

[31]   De Sousa E Melo F, Vermeulen L, Fessler E, Medema JP, Medema JP. Cancer heterogeneity--a multifaceted view. EMBO Rep 2013; 14(8): 686-95.

[http://dx.doi.org/10.1038/embor.2013.92] [PMID: 23846313]

[32] Lang F, Wojcik B, Rieger MA. Stem cell hierarchy and clonal evolution in acute lymphoblastic leukemia. Stem Cells Int 2015; 2015: 137164.
[http://dx.doi.org/10.1155/2015/137164] [PMID: 26236346]

[33] Rivera C, Rivera S, Loriot Y, Vozenin MC, Deutsch E. Lung cancer stem cell: New insights on experimental models and preclinical data. J Oncol 2011; 2011: 549181.
[http://dx.doi.org/10.1155/2011/549181] [PMID: 21209720]

[34] Wang W, Quan Y, Fu Q, *et al.* Dynamics between cancer cell subpopulations reveals a model coordinating with both hierarchical and stochastic concepts. PLoS One 2014; 9(1): e84654.
[http://dx.doi.org/10.1371/journal.pone.0084654] [PMID: 24416258]

[35] Song Y, Wang Y, Tong C, *et al.* A unified model of the hierarchical and stochastic theories of gastric cancer. Br J Cancer 2017; 116(8): 973-89.
[http://dx.doi.org/10.1038/bjc.2017.54] [PMID: 28301871]

[36] Lawson DA, Kessenbrock K, Davis RT, Pervolarakis N, Werb Z. Tumour heterogeneity and metastasis at single-cell resolution. Nat Cell Biol 2018; 20(12): 1349-60.
[http://dx.doi.org/10.1038/s41556-018-0236-7] [PMID: 30482943]

[37] Albini A, Bruno A, Gallo C, Pajardi G, Noonan DM, Dallaglio K. Cancer stem cells and the tumor microenvironment: Interplay in tumor heterogeneity. Connect Tissue Res 2015; 56(5): 414-25.
[http://dx.doi.org/10.3109/03008207.2015.1066780] [PMID: 26291921]

[38] Wang A, Chen L, Li C, Zhu Y. Heterogeneity in cancer stem cells. Cancer Lett 2015; 357(1): 63-8.
[http://dx.doi.org/10.1016/j.canlet.2014.11.040] [PMID: 25444897]

[39] Visvader JE, Lindeman GJ. Cancer stem cells: Current status and evolving complexities. Cell Stem Cell 2012; 10(6): 717-28.
[http://dx.doi.org/10.1016/j.stem.2012.05.007] [PMID: 22704512]

[40] Greaves M, Maley CC. Clonal evolution in cancer. Nature 2012; 481(7381): 306-13.
[http://dx.doi.org/10.1038/nature10762] [PMID: 22258609]

[41] Campbell LL, Polyak K. Breast tumor heterogeneity: Cancer stem cells or clonal evolution? Cell Cycle 2007; 6(19): 2332-8.
[http://dx.doi.org/10.4161/cc.6.19.4914] [PMID: 17786053]

[42] Vitale I, Manic G, De Maria R, Kroemer G, Galluzzi L. DNA damage in stem cells. Mol Cell 2017; 66(3): 306-19.
[http://dx.doi.org/10.1016/j.molcel.2017.04.006] [PMID: 28475867]

[43] Wang QE. DNA damage responses in cancer stem cells: Implications for cancer therapeutic strategies. World J Biol Chem 2015; 6(3): 57-64.
[http://dx.doi.org/10.4331/wjbc.v6.i3.57] [PMID: 26322164]

[44] Ceccarelli S, Megiorni F, Bellavia D, Marchese C, Screpanti I, Checquolo S. Notch3 targeting: A novel weapon against ovarian cancer stem cells. Stem Cells Int 2019; 2019: 6264931.
[http://dx.doi.org/10.1155/2019/6264931] [PMID: 30723507]

[45] Katoh M. Networking of WNT, FGF, Notch, BMP, and Hedgehog signaling pathways during carcinogenesis. Stem Cell Rev 2007; 3(1): 30-8.
[http://dx.doi.org/10.1007/s12015-007-0006-6] [PMID: 17873379]

[46] Katoh M, Katoh M. WNT signaling pathway and stem cell signaling network. Clin Cancer Res 2007; 13(14): 4042-5.
[http://dx.doi.org/10.1158/1078-0432.CCR-06-2316] [PMID: 17634527]

[47] Pan T, Xu J, Zhu Y. Self-renewal molecular mechanisms of colorectal cancer stem cells. Int J Mol Med 2017; 39(1): 9-20.
[http://dx.doi.org/10.3892/ijmm.2016.2815] [PMID: 27909729]

[48]   Zaravinos A. The regulatory role of microRNAs in EMT and cancer. J Oncol 2015; 2015: 865816.
        [http://dx.doi.org/10.1155/2015/865816] [PMID: 25883654]

[49]   Czerwinska P, Kaminska B. Regulation of breast cancer stem cell features. Contemp Oncol (Pozn)
        2015; 19(1A): A7-A15.
        [http://dx.doi.org/10.5114/wo.2014.47126] [PMID: 25691826]

[50]   Mani SA, Guo W, Liao MJ, *et al.* The epithelial-mesenchymal transition generates cells with
        properties of stem cells. Cell 2008; 133(4): 704-15.
        [http://dx.doi.org/10.1016/j.cell.2008.03.027] [PMID: 18485877]

[51]   Brinckerhoff CE. Cancer Stem Cells (CSCs) in melanoma: There's smoke, but is there fire? J Cell
        Physiol 2017; 232(10): 2674-8.
        [http://dx.doi.org/10.1002/jcp.25796] [PMID: 28078710]

[52]   Teng YD, Wang L, Kabatas S, Ulrich H, Zafonte RD. Cancer stem cells or tumor survival cells? Stem
        Cells Dev 2018; 27(21): 1466-78.
        [http://dx.doi.org/10.1089/scd.2018.0129] [PMID: 30092726]

[53]   Bonnet D, Dick JE. Human acute myeloid leukemia is organized as a hierarchy that originates from a
        primitive hematopoietic cell. Nat Med 1997; 3(7): 730-7.
        [http://dx.doi.org/10.1038/nm0797-730] [PMID: 9212098]

[54]   Jin X, Jin X, Kim H. Cancer stem cells and differentiation therapy. Tumour Biol 2017; 39(10):
        1010428317729933.
        [http://dx.doi.org/10.1177/1010428317729933] [PMID: 29072131]

[55]   Sainz B Jr, Carron E, Vallespinós M, Machado HL. Cancer stem cells and macrophages: Implications
        in tumor biology and therapeutic strategies. Mediators Inflamm 2016; 2016: 9012369.
        [http://dx.doi.org/10.1155/2016/9012369] [PMID: 26980947]

[56]   Nio K, Yamashita T, Kaneko S. The evolving concept of liver cancer stem cells. Mol Cancer 2017;
        16(1): 4-15.
        [http://dx.doi.org/10.1186/s12943-016-0572-9] [PMID: 28137313]

[57]   Gerber JM, Smith BD, Ngwang B, *et al.* A clinically relevant population of leukemic CD34(+)CD38(-
) cells in acute myeloid leukemia. Blood 2012; 119(15): 3571-7.
        [http://dx.doi.org/10.1182/blood-2011-06-364182] [PMID: 22262762]

[58]   Shao J, Fan W, Ma B, Wu Y. Breast cancer stem cells expressing different stem cell markers exhibit
        distinct biological characteristics. Mol Med Rep 2016; 14(6): 4991-8.
        [http://dx.doi.org/10.3892/mmr.2016.5899] [PMID: 27840965]

[59]   Cheng JX, Liu BL, Zhang X. How powerful is CD133 as a cancer stem cell marker in brain tumors?
        Cancer Treat Rev 2009; 35(5): 403-8.
        [http://dx.doi.org/10.1016/j.ctrv.2009.03.002] [PMID: 19369008]

[60]   Gao M, Kong Y, Yang G, Gao L, Shi J. Multiple myeloma cancer stem cells. Oncotarget 2016; 7(23):
        35466-77.
        [http://dx.doi.org/10.18632/oncotarget.8154] [PMID: 27007154]

[61]   Ishiwata T, Matsuda Y, Yoshimura H, *et al.* Pancreatic cancer stem cells: Features and detection
        methods. Pathol Oncol Res 2018; 24(4): 797-805.
        [http://dx.doi.org/10.1007/s12253-018-0420-x] [PMID: 29948612]

[62]   Han J, Fujisawa T, Husain SR, Puri RK. Identification and characterization of cancer stem cells in
        human head and neck squamous cell carcinoma. BMC Cancer 2014; 14: 173-83.
        [http://dx.doi.org/10.1186/1471-2407-14-173] [PMID: 24612587]

[63]   Ren F, Sheng WQ, Du X. CD133: A cancer stem cells marker, is used in colorectal cancers. World J
        Gastroenterol 2013; 19(17): 2603-11.
        [http://dx.doi.org/10.3748/wjg.v19.i17.2603] [PMID: 23674867]

[64]   Sun JH, Luo Q, Liu LL, Song GB. Liver cancer stem cell markers: Progression and therapeutic implications. World J Gastroenterol 2016; 22(13): 3547-57.
[http://dx.doi.org/10.3748/wjg.v22.i13.3547] [PMID: 27053846]

[65]   Wang S, Xu ZY, Wang LF, Su W. CD133⁺ cancer stem cells in lung cancer. Front Biosci 2013; 18: 447-53.
[http://dx.doi.org/10.2741/4113] [PMID: 23276935]

[66]   Chen J, Wang J, Chen D, *et al.* Evaluation of characteristics of CD44⁺CD117⁺ ovarian cancer stem cells in three dimensional basement membrane extract scaffold versus two dimensional monocultures. BMC Cell Biol 2013; 14: 7-17.
[http://dx.doi.org/10.1186/1471-2121-14-7] [PMID: 23368632]

[67]   Güler G, Guven U, Oktem G. Characterization of CD133⁺/CD44⁺ human prostate cancer stem cells with ATR-FTIR spectroscopy. Analyst (Lond) 2019; 144(6): 2138-49.
[http://dx.doi.org/10.1039/C9AN00093C] [PMID: 30742170]

[68]   S Franco S, Szczesna K, Iliou MS, *et al. In vitro* models of cancer stem cells and clinical applications. BMC Cancer 2016; 16(Suppl. 2): 738-64.
[http://dx.doi.org/10.1186/s12885-016-2774-3] [PMID: 27766946]

[69]   Bentivegna A, Conconi D, Panzeri E, *et al.* Biological heterogeneity of putative bladder cancer stem-like cell populations from human bladder transitional cell carcinoma samples. Cancer Sci 2010; 101(2): 416-24.
[http://dx.doi.org/10.1111/j.1349-7006.2009.01414.x] [PMID: 19961489]

[70]   Masuko K, Okazaki S, Satoh M, *et al.* Anti-tumor effect against human cancer xenografts by a fully human monoclonal antibody to a variant 8-epitope of CD44R1 expressed on cancer stem cells. PLoS One 2012; 7(1): e29728.
[http://dx.doi.org/10.1371/journal.pone.0029728] [PMID: 22272243]

[71]   Singh SK, Clarke ID, Terasaki M, *et al.* Identification of a cancer stem cell in human brain tumors. Cancer Res 2003; 63(18): 5821-8.
[PMID: 14522905]

[72]   Al-Hajj M, Wicha MS, Benito-Hernandez A, Morrison SJ, Clarke MF. Prospective identification of tumorigenic breast cancer cells. Proc Natl Acad Sci USA 2003; 100(7): 3983-8.
[http://dx.doi.org/10.1073/pnas.0530291100] [PMID: 12629218]

[73]   Bao S, Wu Q, Li Z, *et al.* Targeting cancer stem cells through L1CAM suppresses glioma growth. Cancer Res 2008; 68(15): 6043-8.
[http://dx.doi.org/10.1158/0008-5472.CAN-08-1079] [PMID: 18676824]

[74]   Fan F, Bellister S, Lu J, *et al.* The requirement for freshly isolated human colorectal cancer (CRC) cells in isolating CRC stem cells. Br J Cancer 2015; 112(3): 539-46.
[http://dx.doi.org/10.1038/bjc.2014.620] [PMID: 25535733]

[75]   Ricci-Vitiani L, Lombardi DG, Pilozzi E, *et al.* Identification and expansion of human colon-cancer-initiating cells. Nature 2007; 445(7123): 111-5.
[http://dx.doi.org/10.1038/nature05384] [PMID: 17122771]

[76]   Takaishi S, Okumura T, Tu S, *et al.* Identification of gastric cancer stem cells using the cell surface marker CD44. Stem Cells 2009; 27(5): 1006-20.
[http://dx.doi.org/10.1002/stem.30] [PMID: 19415765]

[77]   Shi C, Tian R, Wang M, *et al.* CD44⁺ CD133⁺ population exhibits cancer stem cell-like characteristics in human gallbladder carcinoma. Cancer Biol Ther 2010; 10(11): 1182-90.
[http://dx.doi.org/10.4161/cbt.10.11.13664] [PMID: 20948317]

[78]   Manohar R, Li Y, Fohrer H, *et al.* Identification of a candidate stem cell in human gallbladder. Stem Cell Res (Amst) 2015; 14(3): 258-69.
[http://dx.doi.org/10.1016/j.scr.2014.12.003] [PMID: 25765520]

[79]   Prince ME, Sivanandan R, Kaczorowski A, *et al.* Identification of a subpopulation of cells with cancer stem cell properties in head and neck squamous cell carcinoma. Proc Natl Acad Sci USA 2007; 104(3): 973-8.
[http://dx.doi.org/10.1073/pnas.0610117104] [PMID: 17210912]

[80]   Yuan ZX, Mo J, Zhao G, Shu G, Fu HL, Zhao W. Targeting strategies for renal cell carcinoma: From renal cancer cells to renal cancer stem cells. Front Pharmacol 2016; 7(423): 423.
[http://dx.doi.org/10.3389/fphar.2016.00423] [PMID: 27891093]

[81]   Hosen N, Park CY, Tatsumi N, *et al.* CD96 is a leukemic stem cell-specific marker in human acute myeloid leukemia. Proc Natl Acad Sci USA 2007; 104(26): 11008-13.
[http://dx.doi.org/10.1073/pnas.0704271104] [PMID: 17576927]

[82]   van Rhenen A, van Dongen GA, Kelder A, *et al.* The novel AML stem cell associated antigen CLL-1 aids in discrimination between normal and leukemic stem cells. Blood 2007; 110(7): 2659-66.
[http://dx.doi.org/10.1182/blood-2007-03-083048] [PMID: 17609428]

[83]   Zeng SS, Yamashita T, Kondo M, *et al.* The transcription factor SALL4 regulates stemness of EpCAM-positive hepatocellular carcinoma. J Hepatol 2014; 60(1): 127-34.
[http://dx.doi.org/10.1016/j.jhep.2013.08.024] [PMID: 24012616]

[84]   Yang ZF, Ho DW, Ng MN, *et al.* Significance of CD90$^+$ cancer stem cells in human liver cancer. Cancer Cell 2008; 13(2): 153-66.
[http://dx.doi.org/10.1016/j.ccr.2008.01.013] [PMID: 18242515]

[85]   Hu Y, Fu L. Targeting cancer stem cells: A new therapy to cure cancer patients. Am J Cancer Res 2012; 2(3): 340-56.
[PMID: 22679565]

[86]   Kumar D, Gorain M, Kundu G, Kundu GC. Therapeutic implications of cellular and molecular biology of cancer stem cells in melanoma. Mol Cancer 2017; 16(1): 7-24.
[http://dx.doi.org/10.1186/s12943-016-0578-3] [PMID: 28137308]

[87]   Schatton T, Murphy GF, Frank NY, *et al.* Identification of cells initiating human melanomas. Nature 2008; 451(7176): 345-9.
[http://dx.doi.org/10.1038/nature06489] [PMID: 18202660]

[88]   Matsui W, Huff CA, Wang Q, *et al.* Characterization of clonogenic multiple myeloma cells. Blood 2004; 103(6): 2332-6.
[http://dx.doi.org/10.1182/blood-2003-09-3064] [PMID: 14630803]

[89]   Matsui W, Wang Q, Barber JP, *et al.* Clonogenic multiple myeloma progenitors, stem cell properties, and drug resistance. Cancer Res 2008; 68(1): 190-7.
[http://dx.doi.org/10.1158/0008-5472.CAN-07-3096] [PMID: 18172311]

[90]   Ming XY, Fu L, Zhang LY, *et al.* Integrin α7 is a functional cancer stem cell surface marker in oesophageal squamous cell carcinoma. Nat Commun 2016; 7(13568): 13568.
[http://dx.doi.org/10.1038/ncomms13568] [PMID: 27924820]

[91]   Zhao JS, Li WJ, Ge D, *et al.* Tumor initiating cells in esophageal squamous cell carcinomas express high levels of CD44. PLoS One 2011; 6(6): e21419.
[http://dx.doi.org/10.1371/journal.pone.0021419] [PMID: 21731740]

[92]   Foster R, Buckanovich RJ, Rueda BR. Ovarian cancer stem cells: Working towards the root of stemness. Cancer Lett 2013; 338(1): 147-57.
[http://dx.doi.org/10.1016/j.canlet.2012.10.023] [PMID: 23138176]

[93]   Skubitz AP, Taras EP, Boylan KL, *et al.* Targeting CD133 in an *in vivo* ovarian cancer model reduces ovarian cancer progression. Gynecol Oncol 2013; 130(3): 579-87.
[http://dx.doi.org/10.1016/j.ygyno.2013.05.027] [PMID: 23721800]

[94]   Li C, Heidt DG, Dalerba P, *et al.* Identification of pancreatic cancer stem cells. Cancer Res 2007;

67(3): 1030-7.
[http://dx.doi.org/10.1158/0008-5472.CAN-06-2030] [PMID: 17283135]

[95]   Li L, Hao X, Qin J, *et al.* Antibody against CD44s inhibits pancreatic tumor initiation and postradiation recurrence in mice. Gastroenterology 2014; 146(4): 1108-18.
[http://dx.doi.org/10.1053/j.gastro.2013.12.035] [PMID: 24397969]

[96]   Chen X, Li Q, Liu X, *et al.* Defining a population of stem-like human prostate cancer cells that can generate and propagate castration-resistant prostate cancer. Clin Cancer Res 2016; 22(17): 4505-16.
[http://dx.doi.org/10.1158/1078-0432.CCR-15-2956] [PMID: 27060154]

[97]   Moltzahn F, Thalmann GN. Cancer stem cells in prostate cancer. Transl Androl Urol 2013; 2(3): 242-53.
[http://dx.doi.org/10.3978/j.issn.2223-4683.2013.09.06] [PMID: 26816738]

[98]   Stratford EW, Bostad M, Castro R, *et al.* Photochemical internalization of CD133-targeting immunotoxins efficiently depletes sarcoma cells with stem-like properties and reduces tumorigenicity. Biochim Biophys Acta 2013; 1830(8): 4235-43.
[http://dx.doi.org/10.1016/j.bbagen.2013.04.033] [PMID: 23643966]

[99]   Edris B, Weiskopf K, Volkmer AK, *et al.* Antibody therapy targeting the CD47 protein is effective in a model of aggressive metastatic leiomyosarcoma. Proc Natl Acad Sci USA 2012; 109(17): 6656-61.
[http://dx.doi.org/10.1073/pnas.1121629109] [PMID: 22451919]

[100]   Nagayama Y, Shimamura M, Mitsutake N. Cancer stem cells in the thyroid. Front Endocrinol (Lausanne) 2016; 7(20): 20.
[http://dx.doi.org/10.3389/fendo.2016.00020] [PMID: 26973599]

[101]   Dong P, Kaneuchi M, Konno Y, Watari H, Sudo S, Sakuragi N. Emerging therapeutic biomarkers in endometrial cancer. BioMed Res Int 2013; 2013: 130362.
[http://dx.doi.org/10.1155/2013/130362] [PMID: 23819113]

[102]   van Niekerk G, Davids LM, Hattingh SM, Engelbrecht AM. Cancer stem cells: A product of clonal evolution? Int J Cancer 2017; 140(5): 993-9.
[http://dx.doi.org/10.1002/ijc.30448] [PMID: 27676693]

[103]   Howard CM, Valluri J, Alberico A, *et al.* Analysis of chemopredictive assay for targeting cancer stem cells in glioblastoma patients. Transl Oncol 2017; 10(2): 241-54.
[http://dx.doi.org/10.1016/j.tranon.2017.01.008] [PMID: 28199863]

[104]   Nassar D, Blanpain C. Cancer stem cells: Basic concepts and therapeutic implications. Annu Rev Pathol 2016; 11: 47-76.
[http://dx.doi.org/10.1146/annurev-pathol-012615-044438] [PMID: 27193450]

[105]   Phi LTH, Sari IN, Yang YG, *et al.* Cancer Stem Cells (CSCs) in drug resistance and their therapeutic implications in cancer treatment. Stem Cells Int 2018; 2018: 5416923.
[http://dx.doi.org/10.1155/2018/5416923] [PMID: 29681949]

[106]   Di C, Zhao Y. Multiple drug resistance due to resistance to stem cells and stem cell treatment progress in cancer (Review). Exp Ther Med 2015; 9(2): 289-93.
[http://dx.doi.org/10.3892/etm.2014.2141] [PMID: 25574188]

[107]   Zhao J. Cancer stem cells and chemoresistance: The smartest survives the raid. Pharmacol Ther 2016; 160: 145-58.
[http://dx.doi.org/10.1016/j.pharmthera.2016.02.008] [PMID: 26899500]

[108]   Pal A, Valdez KE, Carletti MZ, Behbod F. Targeting the perpetrator: Breast cancer stem cell therapeutics. Curr Drug Targets 2010; 11(9): 1147-56.
[http://dx.doi.org/10.2174/138945010792006843] [PMID: 20545606]

[109]   Takeishi S, Nakayama KI. To wake up cancer stem cells, or to let them sleep, that is the question. Cancer Sci 2016; 107(7): 875-81.
[http://dx.doi.org/10.1111/cas.12958] [PMID: 27116333]

[110] Moselhy J, Srinivasan S, Ankem MK, Damodaran C. Natural products that target cancer stem cells. Anticancer Res 2015; 35(11): 5773-88.
[PMID: 26503998]

[111] Faurobert E, Bouin AP, Albiges-Rizo C. Microenvironment, tumor cell plasticity, and cancer. Curr Opin Oncol 2015; 27(1): 64-70.
[http://dx.doi.org/10.1097/CCO.0000000000000154] [PMID: 25415136]

[112] Park JH, Chung S, Matsuo Y, Nakamura Y. Development of small molecular compounds targeting cancer stem cells. MedChemComm 2016; 8(1): 73-80.
[http://dx.doi.org/10.1039/C6MD00385K] [PMID: 30108692]

[113] Wang A, Qu L, Wang L. At the crossroads of cancer stem cells and targeted therapy resistance. Cancer Lett 2017; 385: 87-96.
[http://dx.doi.org/10.1016/j.canlet.2016.10.039] [PMID: 27816488]

[114] Kim WT, Ryu CJ. Cancer stem cell surface markers on normal stem cells. BMB Rep 2017; 50(6): 285-98.
[http://dx.doi.org/10.5483/BMBRep.2017.50.6.039] [PMID: 28270302]

[115] Alison MR, Lim SM, Nicholson LJ. Cancer stem cells: Problems for therapy? J Pathol 2011; 223(2): 147-61.
[http://dx.doi.org/10.1002/path.2793] [PMID: 21125672]

[116] Weiswald LB, Bellet D, Dangles-Marie V. Spherical cancer models in tumor biology. Neoplasia 2015; 17(1): 1-15.
[http://dx.doi.org/10.1016/j.neo.2014.12.004] [PMID: 25622895]

[117] Han L, Shi S, Gong T, Zhang Z, Sun X. Cancer stem cells: Therapeutic implications and perspectives in cancer therapy. Acta Pharm Sin B 2013; 3(2): 65-75.
[http://dx.doi.org/10.1016/j.apsb.2013.02.006]

[118] Gilbert CA, Ross AH. Cancer stem cells: Cell culture, markers, and targets for new therapies. J Cell Biochem 2009; 108(5): 1031-8.
[http://dx.doi.org/10.1002/jcb.22350] [PMID: 19760641]

[119] Pastrana E, Silva-Vargas V, Doetsch F. Eyes wide open: A critical review of sphere-formation as an assay for stem cells. Cell Stem Cell 2011; 8(5): 486-98.
[http://dx.doi.org/10.1016/j.stem.2011.04.007] [PMID: 21549325]

[120] Lonardo E, Cioffi M, Sancho P, Crusz S, Heeschen C. Studying pancreatic cancer stem cell characteristics for developing new treatment strategies. J Vis Exp 2015; 100(100): e52801.
[http://dx.doi.org/10.3791/52801] [PMID: 26132091]

[121] Abbas H, Elyamany A, Salem M, Salem A, Binziad S, Gamal B. The optimal sequence of radiotherapy and chemotherapy in adjuvant treatment of breast cancer. Int Arch Med 2011; 4(1): 35-41.
[http://dx.doi.org/10.1186/1755-7682-4-35] [PMID: 21999819]

[122] Ranjan T, Abrey LE. Current management of metastatic brain disease. Neurotherapeutics 2009; 6(3): 598-603.
[http://dx.doi.org/10.1016/j.nurt.2009.04.012] [PMID: 19560748]

[123] Zappa C, Mousa SA. Non-small cell lung cancer: Current treatment and future advances. Transl Lung Cancer Res 2016; 5(3): 288-300.
[http://dx.doi.org/10.21037/tlcr.2016.06.07] [PMID: 27413711]

[124] Fields EC, McGuire WP, Lin L, Temkin SM. Radiation treatment in women with ovarian cancer: Past, present, and future. Front Oncol 2017; 7(177): 177.
[http://dx.doi.org/10.3389/fonc.2017.00177] [PMID: 28871275]

[125] Häfner MF, Debus J. Radiotherapy for colorectal cancer: Current standards and future perspectives.

Visc Med 2016; 32(3): 172-7.
[http://dx.doi.org/10.1159/000446486] [PMID: 27493944]

[126] Baskar R, Lee KA, Yeo R, Yeoh KW. Cancer and radiation therapy: Current advances and future directions. Int J Med Sci 2012; 9(3): 193-9.
[http://dx.doi.org/10.7150/ijms.3635] [PMID: 22408567]

[127] Ramirez LY, Huestis SE, Yap TY, Zyzanski S, Drotar D, Kodish E. Potential chemotherapy side effects: What do oncologists tell parents? Pediatr Blood Cancer 2009; 52(4): 497-502.
[http://dx.doi.org/10.1002/pbc.21835] [PMID: 19101994]

[128] Liu Z, Huang P, Law S, Tian H, Leung W, Xu C. Preventive effect of curcumin against chemotherapy-induced side-effects. Front Pharmacol 2018; 9(1374): 1374.
[http://dx.doi.org/10.3389/fphar.2018.01374] [PMID: 30538634]

[129] Arruebo M, Vilaboa N, Sáez-Gutierrez B, *et al.* Assessment of the evolution of cancer treatment therapies. Cancers (Basel) 2011; 3(3): 3279-330.
[http://dx.doi.org/10.3390/cancers3033279] [PMID: 24212956]

[130] Bagnyukova TV, Serebriiskii IG, Zhou Y, Hopper-Borge EA, Golemis EA, Astsaturov I. Chemotherapy and signaling: How can targeted therapies supercharge cytotoxic agents? Cancer Biol Ther 2010; 10(9): 839-53.
[http://dx.doi.org/10.4161/cbt.10.9.13738] [PMID: 20935499]

[131] Moitra K, Lou H, Dean M. Multidrug efflux pumps and cancer stem cells: Insights into multidrug resistance and therapeutic development. Clin Pharmacol Ther 2011; 89(4): 491-502.
[http://dx.doi.org/10.1038/clpt.2011.14] [PMID: 21368752]

[132] Vander Linden C, Corbet C. Therapeutic targeting of cancer stem cells: Integrating and exploiting the acidic niche. Front Oncol 2019; 9(159): 159.
[http://dx.doi.org/10.3389/fonc.2019.00159] [PMID: 30941310]

[133] Oei AL, Vriend LEM, Krawczyk PM, Horsman MR, Franken NAP, Crezee J. Targeting therapy-resistant cancer stem cells by hyperthermia. Int J Hyperthermia 2017; 33(4): 419-27.
[http://dx.doi.org/10.1080/02656736.2017.1279757] [PMID: 28100096]

[134] Jiang WG, Sanders AJ, Katoh M, *et al.* Tissue invasion and metastasis: Molecular, biological and clinical perspectives. Semin Cancer Biol 2015; 35(Suppl.): S244-75.
[http://dx.doi.org/10.1016/j.semcancer.2015.03.008] [PMID: 25865774]

[135] Yakisich JS. System models, assays and endpoint parameters to evaluate anticancer compounds during preclinical screening. Curr Med Chem 2014; 21(35): 3985-98.
[http://dx.doi.org/10.2174/09298673113209990009] [PMID: 23701499]

[136] Evans JM, Donnelly LA, Emslie-Smith AM, Alessi DR, Morris AD. Metformin and reduced risk of cancer in diabetic patients. BMJ 2005; 330(7503): 1304-5.
[http://dx.doi.org/10.1136/bmj.38415.708634.F7] [PMID: 15849206]

[137] Saini N, Yang X. Metformin as an anti-cancer agent: Actions and mechanisms targeting cancer stem cells. Acta Biochim Biophys Sin (Shanghai) 2018; 50(2): 133-43.
[http://dx.doi.org/10.1093/abbs/gmx106] [PMID: 29342230]

[138] Liu H, Lv L, Yang K. Chemotherapy targeting cancer stem cells. Am J Cancer Res 2015; 5(3): 880-93.
[PMID: 26045975]

[139] Fletcher JI, Haber M, Henderson MJ, Norris MD. ABC transporters in cancer: More than just drug efflux pumps. Nat Rev Cancer 2010; 10(2): 147-56.
[http://dx.doi.org/10.1038/nrc2789] [PMID: 20075923]

[140] Murota Y, Tabu K, Taga T. Requirement of ABC transporter inhibition and Hoechst 33342 dye deprivation for the assessment of side population-defined C6 glioma stem cell metabolism using fluorescent probes. BMC Cancer 2016; 16(1): 847-53.
[http://dx.doi.org/10.1186/s12885-016-2895-8] [PMID: 27814696]

[141]   Goodell MA, Brose K, Paradis G, Conner AS, Mulligan RC. Isolation and functional properties of murine hematopoietic stem cells that are replicating *in vivo*. J Exp Med 1996; 183(4): 1797-806.
[http://dx.doi.org/10.1084/jem.183.4.1797] [PMID: 8666936]

[142]   Cui H, Zhang AJ, Chen M, Liu JJ. ABC transporter inhibitors in reversing multidrug resistance to chemotherapy. Curr Drug Targets 2015; 16(12): 1356-71.
[http://dx.doi.org/10.2174/1389450116666150330113506] [PMID: 25901528]

[143]   Jaramillo AC, Al Saig F, Cloos J, Jansen G, Peters GJ. How to overcome ATP-binding cassette drug efflux transporter-mediated drug resistance? Cancer Drug Resist 2018; 1(1): 6-29.
[http://dx.doi.org/10.20517/cdr.2018.02]

[144]   Tan B, Piwnica-Worms D, Ratner L. Multidrug resistance transporters and modulation. Curr Opin Oncol 2000; 12(5): 450-8.
[http://dx.doi.org/10.1097/00001622-200009000-00011] [PMID: 10975553]

[145]   Shukla S, Ohnuma S, Ambudkar SV. Improving cancer chemotherapy with modulators of ABC drug transporters. Curr Drug Targets 2011; 12(5): 621-30.
[http://dx.doi.org/10.2174/138945011795378540] [PMID: 21039338]

[146]   Kathawala RJ, Gupta P, Ashby CR Jr, Chen ZS. The modulation of ABC transporter-mediated multidrug resistance in cancer: A review of the past decade. Drug Resist Updat 2015; 18: 1-17.
[http://dx.doi.org/10.1016/j.drup.2014.11.002] [PMID: 25554624]

[147]   Wu CP, Calcagno AM, Ambudkar SV. Reversal of ABC drug transporter-mediated multidrug resistance in cancer cells: Evaluation of current strategies. Curr Mol Pharmacol 2008; 1(2): 93-105.
[http://dx.doi.org/10.2174/1874467210801020093] [PMID: 19079736]

[148]   Cort A, Ozben T. Natural product modulators to overcome multidrug resistance in cancer. Nutr Cancer 2015; 67(3): 411-23.
[http://dx.doi.org/10.1080/01635581.2015.1002624] [PMID: 25649862]

[149]   Tran VH, Marks D, Duke RK, Bebawy M, Duke CC, Roufogalis BD. Modulation of P-glycoprotei-mediated anticancer drug accumulation, cytotoxicity, and ATPase activity by flavonoid interactions. Nutr Cancer 2011; 63(3): 435-43.
[http://dx.doi.org/10.1080/01635581.2011.535959] [PMID: 21462089]

[150]   Bansal T, Jaggi M, Khar RK, Talegaonkar S. Emerging significance of flavonoids as P-glycoprotein inhibitors in cancer chemotherapy. J Pharm Pharm Sci 2009; 12(1): 46-78.
[http://dx.doi.org/10.18433/J3RC77] [PMID: 19470292]

[151]   de Pace RC, Liu X, Sun M, *et al.* Anticancer activities of (-)-epigallocatechin-3-gallate encapsulated nanoliposomes in MCF7 breast cancer cells. J Liposome Res 2013; 23(3): 187-96.
[http://dx.doi.org/10.3109/08982104.2013.788023] [PMID: 23600473]

[152]   Farabegoli F, Papi A, Bartolini G, Ostan R, Orlandi M. (-)-Epigallocatechin-3-gallate downregulates Pg-P and BCRP in a tamoxifen resistant MCF-7 cell line. Phytomedicine 2010; 17(5): 356-62.
[http://dx.doi.org/10.1016/j.phymed.2010.01.001] [PMID: 20149610]

[153]   Qian F, Wei D, Zhang Q, Yang S. Modulation of P-glycoprotein function and reversal of multidrug resistance by (-)-epigallocatechin gallate in human cancer cells. Biomed Pharmacother 2005; 59(3): 64-9.
[http://dx.doi.org/10.1016/j.biopha.2005.01.002] [PMID: 15795098]

[154]   Sreejayan , Rao MN. Nitric oxide scavenging by curcuminoids. J Pharm Pharmacol 1997; 49(1): 105-7.
[http://dx.doi.org/10.1111/j.2042-7158.1997.tb06761.x] [PMID: 9120760]

[155]   Jiang M, Huang O, Zhang X, *et al.* Curcumin induces cell death and restores tamoxifen sensitivity in the antiestrogen-resistant breast cancer cell lines MCF-7/LCC2 and MCF-7/LCC9. Molecules 2013; 18(1): 701-20.
[http://dx.doi.org/10.3390/molecules18010701] [PMID: 23299550]

[156]   Everett PC, Meyers JA, Makkinje A, Rabbi M, Lerner A. Preclinical assessment of curcumin as a potential therapy for B-CLL. Am J Hematol 2007; 82(1): 23-30.
[http://dx.doi.org/10.1002/ajh.20757] [PMID: 16947318]

[157]   Sadzuka Y, Nagamine M, Toyooka T, Ibuki Y, Sonobe T. Beneficial effects of curcumin on antitumor activity and adverse reactions of doxorubicin. Int J Pharm 2012; 432(1-2): 42-9.
[http://dx.doi.org/10.1016/j.ijpharm.2012.04.062] [PMID: 22569233]

[158]   Duarte VM, Han E, Veena MS, *et al.* Curcumin enhances the effect of cisplatin in suppression of head and neck squamous cell carcinoma via inhibition of IKKβ protein of the NFκB pathway. Mol Cancer Ther 2010; 9(10): 2665-75.
[http://dx.doi.org/10.1158/1535-7163.MCT-10-0064] [PMID: 20937593]

[159]   Patel D, Shukla S, Gupta S. Apigenin and cancer chemoprevention: Progress, potential and promise (review). Int J Oncol 2007; 30(1): 233-45.
[http://dx.doi.org/10.3892/ijo.30.1.233] [PMID: 17143534]

[160]   Hashemi M, Nouri Long M, Entezari M, Nafisi S, Nowroozii H. Anti-mutagenic and pro-apoptotic effects of apigenin on human chronic lymphocytic leukemia cells. Acta Med Iran 2010; 48(5): 283-8.
[PMID: 21287458]

[161]   Pang B, Zhao LH, Zhou Q, *et al.* Application of berberine on treating type 2 diabetes mellitus. Int J Endocrinol 2015; 2015: 905749.
[http://dx.doi.org/10.1155/2015/905749] [PMID: 25861268]

[162]   Kumar A, Ekavali , Chopra K, Mukherjee M, Pottabathini R, Dhull DK. Current knowledge and pharmacological profile of berberine: An update. Eur J Pharmacol 2015; 761: 288-97.
[http://dx.doi.org/10.1016/j.ejphar.2015.05.068] [PMID: 26092760]

[163]   Lu B, Hu M, Liu K, Peng J. Cytotoxicity of berberine on human cervical carcinoma HeLa cells through mitochondria, death receptor and MAPK pathways, and *in silico* drug-target prediction. Toxicol In Vitro 2010; 24(6): 1482-90.
[http://dx.doi.org/10.1016/j.tiv.2010.07.017] [PMID: 20656010]

[164]   Park SH, Sung JH, Chung N. Berberine diminishes side population and down-regulates stem cell-associated genes in the pancreatic cancer cell lines PANC-1 and MIA PaCa-2. Mol Cell Biochem 2014; 394(1-2): 209-15.
[http://dx.doi.org/10.1007/s11010-014-2096-1] [PMID: 24894821]

[165]   Ma X, Zhou J, Zhang CX, *et al.* Modulation of drug-resistant membrane and apoptosis proteins of breast cancer stem cells by targeting berberine liposomes. Biomaterials 2013; 34(18): 4452-65.
[http://dx.doi.org/10.1016/j.biomaterials.2013.02.066] [PMID: 23518403]

[166]   Jung SK, Lee MH, Lim DY, *et al.* Isoliquiritigenin induces apoptosis and inhibits xenograft tumor growth of human lung cancer cells by targeting both wild type and L858R/T790M mutant EGFR. J Biol Chem 2014; 289(52): 35839-48.
[http://dx.doi.org/10.1074/jbc.M114.585513] [PMID: 25368326]

[167]   Zheng H, Li Y, Wang Y, *et al.* Downregulation of COX-2 and CYP 4A signaling by isoliquiritigenin inhibits human breast cancer metastasis through preventing anoikis resistance, migration and invasion. Toxicol Appl Pharmacol 2014; 280(1): 10-20.
[http://dx.doi.org/10.1016/j.taap.2014.07.018] [PMID: 25094029]

[168]   Torquato HF, Goettert MI, Justo GZ, Paredes-Gamero EJ. Anti-cancer phytometabolites targeting cancer stem cells. Curr Genomics 2017; 18(2): 156-74.
[http://dx.doi.org/10.2174/1389202917666160803162309] [PMID: 28367074]

[169]   Ayre SG, Perez Garcia y Bellon D, Perez Garcia D Jr. Insulin potentiation therapy: A new concept in the management of chronic degenerative disease. Med Hypotheses 1986; 20(2): 199-210.
[http://dx.doi.org/10.1016/0306-9877(86)90126-X] [PMID: 3526099]

[170]   Malaguarnera R, Belfiore A. The insulin receptor: A new target for cancer therapy. Front Endocrinol

(Lausanne) 2011; 2(93): 93.
[http://dx.doi.org/10.3389/fendo.2011.00093] [PMID: 22654833]

[171]   Malaguarnera R, Belfiore A. The emerging role of insulin and insulin-like growth factor signaling in cancer stem cells. Front Endocrinol (Lausanne) 2014; 5(10): 10.
[http://dx.doi.org/10.3389/fendo.2014.00010] [PMID: 24550888]

[172]   Rostoker R, Abelson S, Bitton-Worms K, *et al.* Highly specific role of the insulin receptor in breast cancer progression. Endocr Relat Cancer 2015; 22(2): 145-57.
[http://dx.doi.org/10.1530/ERC-14-0490] [PMID: 25694511]

[173]   Stoff JA. Selected office based anticancer treatment strategies. J Oncol 2019; 2019: 7462513.
[http://dx.doi.org/10.1155/2019/7462513] [PMID: 30766601]

[174]   Chaffer CL, Brueckmann I, Scheel C, *et al.* Normal and neoplastic nonstem cells can spontaneously convert to a stem-like state. Proc Natl Acad Sci USA 2011; 108(19): 7950-5.
[http://dx.doi.org/10.1073/pnas.1102454108] [PMID: 21498687]

[175]   Zhang D, Tang DG, Rycaj K. Cancer stem cells: Regulation programs, immunological properties and immunotherapy. Semin Cancer Biol 2018; 52(Pt 2): 94-106.
[http://dx.doi.org/10.1016/j.semcancer.2018.05.001] [PMID: 29752993]

[176]   Li Y, Atkinson K, Zhang T. Combination of chemotherapy and cancer stem cell targeting agents: Preclinical and clinical studies. Cancer Lett 2017; 396: 103-9.
[http://dx.doi.org/10.1016/j.canlet.2017.03.008] [PMID: 28300634]

[177]   Dewangan J, Srivastava S, Rath SK. Salinomycin: A new paradigm in cancer therapy. Tumour Biol 2017; 39(3): 1010428317695035.
[http://dx.doi.org/10.1177/1010428317695035] [PMID: 28349817]

[178]   Lu D, Choi MY, Yu J, Castro JE, Kipps TJ, Carson DA. Salinomycin inhibits Wnt signaling and selectively induces apoptosis in chronic lymphocytic leukemia cells. Proc Natl Acad Sci USA 2011; 108(32): 13253-7.
[http://dx.doi.org/10.1073/pnas.1110431108] [PMID: 21788521]

[179]   Wang T, Narayanaswamy R, Ren H, Torchilin VP. Combination therapy targeting both cancer stem-like cells and bulk tumor cells for improved efficacy of breast cancer treatment. Cancer Biol Ther 2016; 17(6): 698-707.
[http://dx.doi.org/10.1080/15384047.2016.1190488] [PMID: 27259361]

[180]   Zhang GN, Liang Y, Zhou LJ, *et al.* Combination of salinomycin and gemcitabine eliminates pancreatic cancer cells. Cancer Lett 2011; 313(2): 137-44.
[http://dx.doi.org/10.1016/j.canlet.2011.05.030] [PMID: 22030254]

[181]   Chen D, Xie F, Sun D, Yin C, Gao J, Zhong Y. Nanomedicine-mediated combination drug therapy in tumor. Open Pharm Sci J 2017; 4: 1-10.
[http://dx.doi.org/10.2174/1874844901704010001]

[182]   Zhang Y, Zhang Q, Sun J, Liu H, Li Q. The combination therapy of salinomycin and gefitinib using poly(d,l-lactic-co-glycolic acid)-poly(ethylene glycol) nanoparticles for targeting both lung cancer stem cells and cancer cells. OncoTargets Ther 2017; 10: 5653-66.
[http://dx.doi.org/10.2147/OTT.S141083] [PMID: 29225473]

[183]   Desai A, Yan Y, Gerson SL. Concise reviews: Cancer stem cell targeted therapies: Toward clinical success. Stem Cells Transl Med 2019; 8(1): 75-81.
[http://dx.doi.org/10.1002/sctm.18-0123] [PMID: 30328686]

[184]   Badrinath N, Yoo SY. Recent advances in cancer stem cell-targeted immunotherapy. Cancers (Basel) 2019; 11(3): 310-23.
[http://dx.doi.org/10.3390/cancers11030310] [PMID: 30841635]

[185]   Schmeel FC, Schmeel LC, Gast SM, Schmidt-Wolf IG. Adoptive immunotherapy strategies with Cytokine-Induced Killer (CIK) cells in the treatment of hematological malignancies. Int J Mol Sci

2014; 15(8): 14632-48.
[http://dx.doi.org/10.3390/ijms150814632] [PMID: 25196601]

[186] Wang X, Tang S, Cui X, *et al.* Cytokine-induced killer cell/dendritic cell-cytokine-induced killer cell immunotherapy for the postoperative treatment of gastric cancer: A systematic review and meta-analysis. Medicine (Baltimore) 2018; 97(36): e12230.
[http://dx.doi.org/10.1097/MD.0000000000012230] [PMID: 30200148]

[187] Vivier E, Raulet DH, Moretta A, *et al.* Innate or adaptive immunity? The example of natural killer cells. Science 2011; 331(6013): 44-9.
[http://dx.doi.org/10.1126/science.1198687] [PMID: 21212348]

[188] Castriconi R, Daga A, Dondero A, *et al.* NK cells recognize and kill human glioblastoma cells with stem cell-like properties. J Immunol 2009; 182(6): 3530-9.
[http://dx.doi.org/10.4049/jimmunol.0802845] [PMID: 19265131]

[189] Dai C, Lin F, Geng R, *et al.* Implication of combined PD-L1/PD-1 blockade with cytokine-induced killer cells as a synergistic immunotherapy for gastrointestinal cancer. Oncotarget 2016; 7(9): 10332-44.
[http://dx.doi.org/10.18632/oncotarget.7243] [PMID: 26871284]

[190] Palucka K, Banchereau J. Cancer immunotherapy via dendritic cells. Nat Rev Cancer 2012; 12(4): 265-77.
[http://dx.doi.org/10.1038/nrc3258] [PMID: 22437871]

[191] Dashti A, Ebrahimi M, Hadjati J, Memarnejadian A, Moazzeni SM. Dendritic cell based immunotherapy using tumor stem cells mediates potent antitumor immune responses. Cancer Lett 2016; 374(1): 175-85.
[http://dx.doi.org/10.1016/j.canlet.2016.01.021] [PMID: 26803056]

[192] Teitz-Tennenbaum S, Wicha MS, Chang AE, Li Q. Targeting cancer stem cells via dendritic-cell vaccination. OncoImmunology 2012; 1(8): 1401-3.
[http://dx.doi.org/10.4161/onci.21026] [PMID: 23243607]

[193] Chen HC, Joalland N, Bridgeman JS, *et al.* Synergistic targeting of breast cancer stem-like cells by human γδ T cells and CD8+ T cells. Immunol Cell Biol 2017; 95(7): 620-9.
[http://dx.doi.org/10.1038/icb.2017.21] [PMID: 28356569]

[194] Miyamoto S, Kochin V, Kanaseki T, *et al.* The antigen ASB4 on cancer stem cells serves as a target for CTL immunotherapy of colorectal cancer. Cancer Immunol Res 2018; 6(3): 358-69.
[http://dx.doi.org/10.1158/2326-6066.CIR-17-0518] [PMID: 29371260]

[195] Hong IS, Jang GB, Lee HY, Nam JS. Targeting cancer stem cells by using the nanoparticles. Int J Nanomedicine 2015; 10(Spec Iss): 251-60.
[http://dx.doi.org/10.2147/IJN.S88310] [PMID: 26425092]

[196] Banerjee ER. Perspectives in Translational Research in Life Sciences and Biomedicine: Translational Outcomes Research in Life Sciences and Translational Medicine. 1st ed. India: Springer 2016.
[http://dx.doi.org/10.1007/978-981-10-0989-1]

[197] Liu R, Kay BK, Jiang S, Chen S. Nanoparticle delivery: Targeting and nonspecific binding. MRS Bull 2009; 34(6): 432-40.
[http://dx.doi.org/10.1557/mrs2009.119]

[198] Friedman AD, Claypool SE, Liu R. The smart targeting of nanoparticles. Curr Pharm Des 2013; 19(35): 6315-29.
[http://dx.doi.org/10.2174/13816128113199990375] [PMID: 23470005]

[199] Yoo J, Park C, Yi G, Lee D, Koo H. Active targeting strategies using biological ligands for nanoparticle drug delivery systems. Cancers (Basel) 2019; 11(5): 640-52.
[http://dx.doi.org/10.3390/cancers11050640] [PMID: 31072061]

[200] Qin W, Huang G, Chen Z, Zhang Y. Nanomaterials in targeting cancer stem cells for cancer therapy.

Front Pharmacol 2017; 8(1): 1-15.
[http://dx.doi.org/10.3389/fphar.2017.00001] [PMID: 28149278]

[201] Asghari F, Khademi R, Esmaeili Ranjbar F, Veisi Malekshahi Z, Faridi Majidi R. Application of nanotechnology in targeting of cancer stem cells: A review. Int J Stem Cells 2019; 12(2): 227-39.
[http://dx.doi.org/10.15283/ijsc19006] [PMID: 31242721]

[202] Jabir NR, Tabrez S, Ashraf GM, Shakil S, Damanhouri GA, Kamal MA. Nanotechnology-based approaches in anticancer research. Int J Nanomedicine 2012; 7: 4391-408.
[http://dx.doi.org/10.2147/IJN.S33838] [PMID: 22927757]

[203] Whitesides GM, Mathias JP, Seto CT. Molecular self-assembly and nanochemistry: A chemical strategy for the synthesis of nanostructures. Science 1991; 254(5036): 1312-9.
[http://dx.doi.org/10.1126/science.1962191] [PMID: 1962191]

[204] Shah V, Taratula O, Garbuzenko OB, Taratula OR, Rodriguez-Rodriguez L, Minko T. Targeted nanomedicine for suppression of CD44 and simultaneous cell death induction in ovarian cancer: An optimal delivery of siRNA and anticancer drug. Clin Cancer Res 2013; 19(22): 6193-204.
[http://dx.doi.org/10.1158/1078-0432.CCR-13-1536] [PMID: 24036854]

[205] Wang L, Su W, Liu Z, *et al.* CD44 antibody-targeted liposomal nanoparticles for molecular imaging and therapy of hepatocellular carcinoma. Biomaterials 2012; 33(20): 5107-14.
[http://dx.doi.org/10.1016/j.biomaterials.2012.03.067] [PMID: 22494888]

[206] Naujokat C. Monoclonal antibodies against human cancer stem cells. Immunotherapy 2014; 6(3): 290-308.
[http://dx.doi.org/10.2217/imt.14.4] [PMID: 24762074]

[207] Naujokat C, Steinhart R. Salinomycin as a drug for targeting human cancer stem cells. J Biomed Biotechnol 2012; 2012: 950658.
[http://dx.doi.org/10.1155/2012/950658] [PMID: 23251084]

[208] Zhang Q, Shi S, Yen Y, Brown J, Ta JQ, Le AD. A subpopulation of CD133(+) cancer stem-like cells characterized in human oral squamous cell carcinoma confer resistance to chemotherapy. Cancer Lett 2010; 289(2): 151-60.
[http://dx.doi.org/10.1016/j.canlet.2009.08.010] [PMID: 19748175]

[209] Piao LS, Hur W, Kim TK, *et al.* CD133$^+$ liver cancer stem cells modulate radioresistance in human hepatocellular carcinoma. Cancer Lett 2012; 315(2): 129-37.
[http://dx.doi.org/10.1016/j.canlet.2011.10.012] [PMID: 22079466]

[210] Lim KJ, Bisht S, Bar EE, Maitra A, Eberhart CG. A polymeric nanoparticle formulation of curcumin inhibits growth, clonogenicity and stem-like fraction in malignant brain tumors. Cancer Biol Ther 2011; 11(5): 464-73.
[http://dx.doi.org/10.4161/cbt.11.5.14410] [PMID: 21193839]

[211] Ni M, Xiong M, Zhang X, *et al.* Poly(lactic-co-glycolic acid) nanoparticles conjugated with CD133 aptamers for targeted salinomycin delivery to CD133$^+$ osteosarcoma cancer stem cells. Int J Nanomedicine 2015; 10: 2537-54.
[http://dx.doi.org/10.2147/IJN.S78498] [PMID: 25848270]

[212] Koppaka V, Thompson DC, Chen Y, *et al.* Aldehyde dehydrogenase inhibitors: A comprehensive review of the pharmacology, mechanism of action, substrate specificity, and clinical application. Pharmacol Rev 2012; 64(3): 520-39.
[http://dx.doi.org/10.1124/pr.111.005538] [PMID: 22544865]

[213] Ma S, Chan KW, Lee TK, *et al.* Aldehyde dehydrogenase discriminates the CD133 liver cancer stem cell populations. Mol Cancer Res 2008; 6(7): 1146-53.
[http://dx.doi.org/10.1158/1541-7786.MCR-08-0035] [PMID: 18644979]

[214] Ginestier C, Hur MH, Charafe-Jauffret E, *et al.* ALDH1 is a marker of normal and malignant human mammary stem cells and a predictor of poor clinical outcome. Cell Stem Cell 2007; 1(5): 555-67.

[http://dx.doi.org/10.1016/j.stem.2007.08.014] [PMID: 18371393]

[215]   Pearce DJ, Taussig D, Simpson C, *et al.* Characterization of cells with a high aldehyde dehydrogenase activity from cord blood and acute myeloid leukemia samples. Stem Cells 2005; 23(6): 752-60.
[http://dx.doi.org/10.1634/stemcells.2004-0292] [PMID: 15917471]

[216]   Rasper M, Schäfer A, Piontek G, *et al.* Aldehyde dehydrogenase 1 positive glioblastoma cells show brain tumor stem cell capacity. Neuro-oncol 2010; 12(10): 1024-33.
[http://dx.doi.org/10.1093/neuonc/noq070] [PMID: 20627895]

[217]   Kuo YC, Wang LJ, Rajesh R. Targeting human brain cancer stem cells by curcumin-loaded nanoparticles grafted with anti-aldehyde dehydrogenase and sialic acid: Colocalization of ALDH and CD44. Mater Sci Eng C 2019; 102: 362-72.
[http://dx.doi.org/10.1016/j.msec.2019.04.065] [PMID: 31147008]

[218]   Chenna V, Hu C, Pramanik D, *et al.* A polymeric nanoparticle encapsulated small-molecule inhibitor of Hedgehog signaling (NanoHHI) bypasses secondary mutational resistance to Smoothened antagonists. Mol Cancer Ther 2012; 11(1): 165-73.
[http://dx.doi.org/10.1158/1535-7163.MCT-11-0341] [PMID: 22027695]

[219]   Yang YM, Chang JW. Bladder Cancer Initiating Cells (BCICs) are among EMA-CD44v6+ subset: Novel methods for isolating undetermined cancer stem (initiating) cells. Cancer Invest 2008; 26(7): 725-33.
[http://dx.doi.org/10.1080/07357900801941845] [PMID: 18608209]

[220]   Huang J, Li C, Wang Y, *et al.* Cytokine-Induced Killer (CIK) cells bound with anti-CD3/anti-CD133 bispecific antibodies target CD133(high) cancer stem cells *in vitro* and *in vivo*. Clin Immunol 2013; 149(1): 156-68.
[http://dx.doi.org/10.1016/j.clim.2013.07.006] [PMID: 23994769]

[221]   Li JF, Niu YY, Xing YL, Liu F. A novel bispecific c-MET/CTLA-4 antibody targetting lung cancer stem cell-like cells with therapeutic potential in human non-small-cell lung cancer. Biosci Rep 2019; 39(5): 1-12.
[http://dx.doi.org/10.1042/BSR20171278] [PMID: 29187584]

[222]   Cooper GM. The Cell: A Molecular Approach. 2nd ed., Sunderland, MA: Sinauer Associates 2000.

[223]   Kumar M, Sharma K, Bhoi S, Kumar M, Pol MM. Expression of p38 mitogen-activated protein kinases, glycogen synthase kinase, c-Jun NH2-terminal kinase, extracellular signal-regulated kinase signaling: Can it be used as molecular markers among trauma-hemorrhagic shock patients? J Emerg Trauma Shock 2016; 9(4): 131-2.
[http://dx.doi.org/10.4103/0974-2700.193346] [PMID: 27904257]

[224]   Wang K, Grivennikov SI, Karin M. Implications of anti-cytokine therapy in colorectal cancer and autoimmune diseases. Ann Rheum Dis 2013; 72(Suppl. 2): ii100-3.
[http://dx.doi.org/10.1136/annrheumdis-2012-202201] [PMID: 23253923]

[225]   Logan CY, Nusse R. The Wnt signaling pathway in development and disease. Annu Rev Cell Dev Biol 2004; 20: 781-810.
[http://dx.doi.org/10.1146/annurev.cellbio.20.010403.113126] [PMID: 15473860]

[226]   MacDonald BT, Tamai K, He X. Wnt/beta-catenin signaling: Components, mechanisms, and diseases. Dev Cell 2009; 17(1): 9-26.
[http://dx.doi.org/10.1016/j.devcel.2009.06.016] [PMID: 19619488]

[227]   Fleming HE, Janzen V, Lo Celso C, *et al.* Wnt signaling in the niche enforces hematopoietic stem cell quiescence and is necessary to preserve self-renewal *in vivo*. Cell Stem Cell 2008; 2(3): 274-83.
[http://dx.doi.org/10.1016/j.stem.2008.01.003] [PMID: 18371452]

[228]   Zhang J, Li Y, Liu Q, Lu W, Bu G. Wnt signaling activation and mammary gland hyperplasia in MMTV-LRP6 transgenic mice: Implication for breast cancer tumorigenesis. Oncogene 2010; 29(4): 539-49.

[http://dx.doi.org/10.1038/onc.2009.339] [PMID: 19881541]

[229] Yallapu MM, Maher DM, Sundram V, Bell MC, Jaggi M, Chauhan SC. Curcumin induces chemo/radio-sensitization in ovarian cancer cells and curcumin nanoparticles inhibit ovarian cancer cell growth. J Ovarian Res 2010; 3(1): 11-22.
[http://dx.doi.org/10.1186/1757-2215-3-11] [PMID: 20429876]

[230] Tang Q, Wang Y, Huang R, *et al.* Preparation of anti-tumor nanoparticle and its inhibition to peritoneal dissemination of colon cancer. PLoS One 2014; 9(6): e98455.
[http://dx.doi.org/10.1371/journal.pone.0098455] [PMID: 24896096]

[231] Segditsas S, Tomlinson I. Colorectal cancer and genetic alterations in the Wnt pathway. Oncogene 2006; 25(57): 7531-7.
[http://dx.doi.org/10.1038/sj.onc.1210059] [PMID: 17143297]

[232] Yin L, Velazquez OC, Liu ZJ. Notch signaling: Emerging molecular targets for cancer therapy. Biochem Pharmacol 2010; 80(5): 690-701.
[http://dx.doi.org/10.1016/j.bcp.2010.03.026] [PMID: 20361945]

[233] Androutsellis-Theotokis A, Leker RR, Soldner F, *et al.* Notch signalling regulates stem cell numbers *in vitro* and *in vivo*. Nature 2006; 442(7104): 823-6.
[http://dx.doi.org/10.1038/nature04940] [PMID: 16799564]

[234] Artavanis-Tsakonas S, Rand MD, Lake RJ. Notch signaling: Cell fate control and signal integration in development. Science 1999; 284(5415): 770-6.
[http://dx.doi.org/10.1126/science.284.5415.770] [PMID: 10221902]

[235] Hovinga KE, Shimizu F, Wang R, *et al.* Inhibition of notch signaling in glioblastoma targets cancer stem cells via an endothelial cell intermediate. Stem Cells 2010; 28(6): 1019-29.
[http://dx.doi.org/10.1002/stem.429] [PMID: 20506127]

[236] Fan X, Khaki L, Zhu TS, *et al.* NOTCH pathway blockade depletes CD133-positive glioblastoma cells and inhibits growth of tumor neurospheres and xenografts. Stem Cells 2010; 28(1): 5-16.
[http://dx.doi.org/10.1002/stem.254] [PMID: 19904829]

[237] Moellering RE, Cornejo M, Davis TN, *et al.* Direct inhibition of the NOTCH transcription factor complex. Nature 2009; 462(7270): 182-8.
[http://dx.doi.org/10.1038/nature08543] [PMID: 19907488]

[238] Mamaeva V, Rosenholm JM, Bate-Eya LT, *et al.* Mesoporous silica nanoparticles as drug delivery systems for targeted inhibition of Notch signaling in cancer. Mol Ther 2011; 19(8): 1538-46.
[http://dx.doi.org/10.1038/mt.2011.105] [PMID: 21629222]

[239] Steg AD, Katre AA, Goodman B, *et al.* Targeting the notch ligand JAGGED1 in both tumor cells and stroma in ovarian cancer. Clin Cancer Res 2011; 17(17): 5674-85.
[http://dx.doi.org/10.1158/1078-0432.CCR-11-0432] [PMID: 21753153]

[240] Itoh S, Itoh F, Goumans MJ, Ten Dijke P. Signaling of transforming growth factor-beta family members through Smad proteins. Eur J Biochem 2000; 267(24): 6954-67.
[http://dx.doi.org/10.1046/j.1432-1327.2000.01828.x] [PMID: 11106403]

[241] Mishra L, Shetty K, Tang Y, Stuart A, Byers SW. The role of TGF-beta and Wnt signaling in gastrointestinal stem cells and cancer. Oncogene 2005; 24(37): 5775-89.
[http://dx.doi.org/10.1038/sj.onc.1208924] [PMID: 16123810]

[242] Liu Z, Bandyopadhyay A, Nichols RW, *et al.* Blockade of autocrine TGF-β signaling inhibits stem cell phenotype, survival, and metastasis of murine breast cancer cells. J Stem Cell Res Ther 2012; 2(1): 1-8.
[http://dx.doi.org/10.4172/2157-7633.1000116] [PMID: 23482850]

[243] Meng H, Zhao Y, Dong J, *et al.* Two-wave nanotherapy to target the stroma and optimize gemcitabine delivery to a human pancreatic cancer model in mice. ACS Nano 2013; 7(11): 10048-65.
[http://dx.doi.org/10.1021/nn404083m] [PMID: 24143858]

[244] Tsai YS, Chen YH, Cheng PC, *et al.* TGF-β1 conjugated to gold nanoparticles results in protein conformational changes and attenuates the biological function. Small 2013; 9(12): 2119-28.
[http://dx.doi.org/10.1002/smll.201202755] [PMID: 23335450]

[245] Villavicencio EH, Walterhouse DO, Iannaccone PM. The sonic hedgehog-patched-Gli pathway in human development and disease. Am J Hum Genet 2000; 67(5): 1047-54.
[http://dx.doi.org/10.1016/S0002-9297(07)62934-6] [PMID: 11001584]

[246] Bai LY, Chiu CF, Lin CW, *et al.* Differential expression of Sonic hedgehog and Gli1 in hematological malignancies. Leukemia 2008; 22(1): 226-8.
[http://dx.doi.org/10.1038/sj.leu.2404978] [PMID: 17928882]

[247] Rubin LL, de Sauvage FJ. Targeting the Hedgehog pathway in cancer. Nat Rev Drug Discov 2006; 5(12): 1026-33.
[http://dx.doi.org/10.1038/nrd2086] [PMID: 17139287]

[248] Ingham PW, McMahon AP. Hedgehog signaling in animal development: Paradigms and principles. Genes Dev 2001; 15(23): 3059-87.
[http://dx.doi.org/10.1101/gad.938601] [PMID: 11731473]

[249] Bhattacharya R, Kwon J, Ali B, *et al.* Role of hedgehog signaling in ovarian cancer. Clin Cancer Res 2008; 14(23): 7659-66.
[http://dx.doi.org/10.1158/1078-0432.CCR-08-1414] [PMID: 19047091]

[250] Park KS, Martelotto LG, Peifer M, *et al.* A crucial requirement for Hedgehog signaling in small cell lung cancer. Nat Med 2011; 17(11): 1504-8.
[http://dx.doi.org/10.1038/nm.2473] [PMID: 21983857]

[251] Xu Y, Chenna V, Hu C, *et al.* Polymeric nanoparticle-encapsulated hedgehog pathway inhibitor HPI-1 (NanoHHI) inhibits systemic metastases in an orthotopic model of human hepatocellular carcinoma. Clin Cancer Res 2012; 18(5): 1291-302.
[http://dx.doi.org/10.1158/1078-0432.CCR-11-0950] [PMID: 21868763]

[252] Verma RK, Yu W, Singh SP, Shankar S, Srivastava RK. Anthothecol-encapsulated PLGA nanoparticles inhibit pancreatic cancer stem cell growth by modulating sonic hedgehog pathway. Nanomedicine (Lond) 2015; 11(8): 2061-70.
[http://dx.doi.org/10.1016/j.nano.2015.07.001] [PMID: 26199979]

[253] Das M, Law S. Role of tumor microenvironment in cancer stem cell chemoresistance and recurrence. Int J Biochem Cell Biol 2018; 103: 115-24.
[http://dx.doi.org/10.1016/j.biocel.2018.08.011] [PMID: 30153480]

[254] Panneerselvam J, Jin J, Shanker M, *et al.* IL-24 inhibits lung cancer cell migration and invasion by disrupting the SDF-1/CXCR4 signaling axis. PLoS One 2015; 10(3): e0122439.
[http://dx.doi.org/10.1371/journal.pone.0122439] [PMID: 25775124]

[255] Orimo A, Gupta PB, Sgroi DC, *et al.* Stromal fibroblasts present in invasive human breast carcinomas promote tumor growth and angiogenesis through elevated SDF-1/CXCL12 secretion. Cell 2005; 121(3): 335-48.
[http://dx.doi.org/10.1016/j.cell.2005.02.034] [PMID: 15882617]

[256] Roma-Rodrigues C, Mendes R, Baptista PV, Fernandes AR. Targeting tumor microenvironment for cancer therapy. Int J Mol Sci 2019; 20(4): 840-70.
[http://dx.doi.org/10.3390/ijms20040840] [PMID: 30781344]

[257] Gun SY, Lee SWL, Sieow JL, Wong SC. Targeting immune cells for cancer therapy. Redox Biol 2019; 25: 101174.
[http://dx.doi.org/10.1016/j.redox.2019.101174] [PMID: 30917934]

[258] Thommen DS, Schumacher TN. T cell dysfunction in cancer. Cancer Cell 2018; 33(4): 547-62.
[http://dx.doi.org/10.1016/j.ccell.2018.03.012] [PMID: 29634943]

[259]   Sanz I, Wei C, Lee FE, Anolik J. Phenotypic and functional heterogeneity of human memory B cells. Semin Immunol 2008; 20(1): 67-82.
[http://dx.doi.org/10.1016/j.smim.2007.12.006] [PMID: 18258454]

[260]   Smith WM, Purvis IJ, Bomstad CN, *et al.* Therapeutic targeting of immune checkpoints with small molecule inhibitors. Am J Transl Res 2019; 11(2): 529-41.
[PMID: 30899360]

[261]   Kather JN, Halama N. Harnessing the innate immune system and local immunological microenvironment to treat colorectal cancer. Br J Cancer 2019; 120(9): 871-82.
[http://dx.doi.org/10.1038/s41416-019-0441-6] [PMID: 30936499]

[262]   Gál P, Varinská L, Fáber L, *et al.* How signaling molecules regulate tumor microenvironment: Parallels to wound repair. Molecules 2017; 22(11): 1818-34.
[http://dx.doi.org/10.3390/molecules22111818] [PMID: 29072623]

[263]   Shin DH, Chun YS, Lee DS, Huang LE, Park JW. Bortezomib inhibits tumor adaptation to hypoxia by stimulating the FIH-mediated repression of hypoxia-inducible factor-1. Blood 2008; 111(6): 3131-6.
[http://dx.doi.org/10.1182/blood-2007-11-120576] [PMID: 18174379]

[264]   Casilli F, Bianchini A, Gloaguen I, *et al.* Inhibition of interleukin-8 (CXCL8/IL-8) responses by repertaxin, a new inhibitor of the chemokine receptors CXCR1 and CXCR2. Biochem Pharmacol 2005; 69(3): 385-94.
[http://dx.doi.org/10.1016/j.bcp.2004.10.007] [PMID: 15652230]

[265]   Welschinger R, Liedtke F, Basnett J, *et al.* Plerixafor (AMD3100) induces prolonged mobilization of acute lymphoblastic leukemia cells and increases the proportion of cycling cells in the blood in mice. Exp Hematol 2013; 41(3): 293-302.e1.
[http://dx.doi.org/10.1016/j.exphem.2012.11.004] [PMID: 23178377]

[266]   Rubin JB, Kung AL, Klein RS, *et al.* A small-molecule antagonist of CXCR4 inhibits intracranial growth of primary brain tumors. Proc Natl Acad Sci USA 2003; 100(23): 13513-8.
[http://dx.doi.org/10.1073/pnas.2235846100] [PMID: 14595012]

[267]   Kajiyama H, Shibata K, Terauchi M, Ino K, Nawa A, Kikkawa F. Involvement of SDF-1alpha/CXCR4 axis in the enhanced peritoneal metastasis of epithelial ovarian carcinoma. Int J Cancer 2008; 122(1): 91-9.
[http://dx.doi.org/10.1002/ijc.23083] [PMID: 17893878]

[268]   Singh B, Cook KR, Martin C, *et al.* Evaluation of a CXCR4 antagonist in a xenograft mouse model of inflammatory breast cancer. Clin Exp Metastasis 2010; 27(4): 233-40.
[http://dx.doi.org/10.1007/s10585-010-9321-4] [PMID: 20229045]

[269]   Drenckhan A, Kurschat N, Dohrmann T, *et al.* Effective inhibition of metastases and primary tumor growth with CTCE-9908 in esophageal cancer. J Surg Res 2013; 182(2): 250-6.
[http://dx.doi.org/10.1016/j.jss.2012.09.035] [PMID: 23117118]

[270]   Wong D, Kandagatla P, Korz W, Chinni SR. Targeting CXCR4 with CTCE-9908 inhibits prostate tumor metastasis. BMC Urol 2014; 14: 12-8.
[http://dx.doi.org/10.1186/1471-2490-14-12] [PMID: 24472670]

[271]   Alphandéry E. Glioblastoma treatments: An account of recent industrial developments. Front Pharmacol 2018; 9(879): 879.
[http://dx.doi.org/10.3389/fphar.2018.00879] [PMID: 30271342]

[272]   Liu SC, Alomran R, Chernikova SB, *et al.* Blockade of SDF-1 after irradiation inhibits tumor recurrences of autochthonous brain tumors in rats. Neuro-oncol 2014; 16(1): 21-8.
[http://dx.doi.org/10.1093/neuonc/not149] [PMID: 24335554]

[273]   Hoellenriegel J, Zboralski D, Maasch C, *et al.* The Spiegelmer NOX-A12, a novel CXCL12 inhibitor, interferes with chronic lymphocytic leukemia cell motility and causes chemosensitization. Blood 2014; 123(7): 1032-9.

[http://dx.doi.org/10.1182/blood-2013-03-493924] [PMID: 24277076]

[274] Burkhardt JK, Hofstetter CP, Santillan A, *et al.* Orthotopic glioblastoma stem-like cell xenograft model in mice to evaluate intra-arterial delivery of bevacizumab: From bedside to bench. J Clin Neurosci 2012; 19(11): 1568-72.
[http://dx.doi.org/10.1016/j.jocn.2012.03.012] [PMID: 22985932]

[275] Prager GW, Poettler M, Unseld M, Zielinski CC. Angiogenesis in cancer: Anti-VEGF escape mechanisms. Transl Lung Cancer Res 2012; 1(1): 14-25.
[PMID: 25806151]

[276] Chiche J, Brahimi-Horn MC, Pouysségur J. Tumour hypoxia induces a metabolic shift causing acidosis: A common feature in cancer. J Cell Mol Med 2010; 14(4): 771-94.
[http://dx.doi.org/10.1111/j.1582-4934.2009.00994.x] [PMID: 20015196]

[277] Wojtkowiak JW, Verduzco D, Schramm KJ, Gillies RJ. Drug resistance and cellular adaptation to tumor acidic pH microenvironment. Mol Pharm 2011; 8(6): 2032-8.
[http://dx.doi.org/10.1021/mp200292c] [PMID: 21981633]

[278] Gatenby RA, Gawlinski ET, Gmitro AF, Kaylor B, Gillies RJ. Acid-mediated tumor invasion: A multidisciplinary study. Cancer Res 2006; 66(10): 5216-23.
[http://dx.doi.org/10.1158/0008-5472.CAN-05-4193] [PMID: 16707446]

[279] Mitra AK, Agrahari V, Mandal A, *et al.* Novel delivery approaches for cancer therapeutics. J Control Release 2015; 219: 248-68.
[http://dx.doi.org/10.1016/j.jconrel.2015.09.067] [PMID: 26456750]

[280] Kydd J, Jadia R, Velpurisiva P, Gad A, Paliwal S, Rai P. Targeting strategies for the combination treatment of cancer using drug delivery systems. Pharmaceutics 2017; 9(4): 46-71.
[http://dx.doi.org/10.3390/pharmaceutics9040046] [PMID: 29036899]

[281] Raucher D, Dragojevic S, Ryu J. Macromolecular drug carriers for targeted glioblastoma therapy: Preclinical studies, challenges, and future perspectives. Front Oncol 2018; 8(624): 624.
[http://dx.doi.org/10.3389/fonc.2018.00624] [PMID: 30619758]

[282] Xu Z, Liu S, Kang Y, Wang M. Glutathione- and pH-responsive nonporous silica prodrug nanoparticles for controlled release and cancer therapy. Nanoscale 2015; 7(13): 5859-68.
[http://dx.doi.org/10.1039/C5NR00297D] [PMID: 25757484]

[283] Xu Z, Wang D, Xu S, Liu X, Zhang X, Zhang H. Preparation of a camptothecin prodrug with glutathione-responsive disulfide linker for anticancer drug delivery. Chem Asian J 2014; 9(1): 199-205.
[http://dx.doi.org/10.1002/asia.201301030] [PMID: 24136878]

[284] Augustine R, Kalva N, Kim HA, Zhang Y, Kim I. pH-Responsive polypeptide-based smart nano-carriers for theranostic applications. Molecules 2019; 24(16): 2961-99.
[http://dx.doi.org/10.3390/molecules24162961] [PMID: 31443287]

[285] Bogen JP, Hinz SC, Grzeschik J, *et al.* Dual function pH responsive bispecific antibodies for tumor targeting and antigen depletion in plasma. Front Immunol 1892; 2019(10): 1892.
[http://dx.doi.org/10.3389/fimmu.2019.01892] [PMID: 31447859]

[286] Zhao Y, Ren W, Zhong T, *et al.* Tumor-specific pH-responsive peptide-modified pH-sensitive liposomes containing doxorubicin for enhancing glioma targeting and anti-tumor activity. J Control Release 2016; 222: 56-66.
[http://dx.doi.org/10.1016/j.jconrel.2015.12.006] [PMID: 26682502]

[287] Ibrahim-Hashim A, Cornnell HH, Abrahams D, *et al.* Systemic buffers inhibit carcinogenesis in TRAMP mice. J Urol 2012; 188(2): 624-31.
[http://dx.doi.org/10.1016/j.juro.2012.03.113] [PMID: 22704445]

[288] Chamie K, Klöpfer P, Bevan P, *et al.* Carbonic anhydrase-IX score is a novel biomarker that predicts recurrence and survival for high-risk, nonmetastatic renal cell carcinoma: Data from the Phase III

ARISER clinical trial. Urol Oncol 2015; 33(5): 204.e25-33.
[http://dx.doi.org/10.1016/j.urolonc.2015.02.013] [PMID: 25823535]

[289] Chekulaeva M, Filipowicz W. Mechanisms of miRNA-mediated post-transcriptional regulation in animal cells. Curr Opin Cell Biol 2009; 21(3): 452-60.
[http://dx.doi.org/10.1016/j.ceb.2009.04.009] [PMID: 19450959]

[290] Chhabra R, Saini N. MicroRNAs in cancer stem cells: Current status and future directions. Tumour Biol 2014; 35(9): 8395-405.
[http://dx.doi.org/10.1007/s13277-014-2264-7] [PMID: 24964962]

[291] Takahashi RU, Miyazaki H, Ochiya T. The role of microRNAs in the regulation of cancer stem cells. Front Genet 2014; 4(295): 295.
[http://dx.doi.org/10.3389/fgene.2013.00295] [PMID: 24427168]

[292] Sethi S, Li Y, Sarkar FH. Regulating miRNA by natural agents as a new strategy for cancer treatment. Curr Drug Targets 2013; 14(10): 1167-74.
[http://dx.doi.org/10.2174/13894501113149990189] [PMID: 23834152]

[293] Aslam MI, Patel M, Singh B, Jameson JS, Pringle JH. MicroRNA manipulation in colorectal cancer cells: From laboratory to clinical application. J Transl Med 2012; 10(128): 128.
[http://dx.doi.org/10.1186/1479-5876-10-128] [PMID: 22716183]

[294] Esau CC. Inhibition of microRNA with antisense oligonucleotides. Methods 2008; 44(1): 55-60.
[http://dx.doi.org/10.1016/j.ymeth.2007.11.001] [PMID: 18158133]

[295] Yu Y, Nangia-Makker P, Farhana L. G Rajendra S, Levi E, Majumdar AP. miR-21 and miR-145 cooperation in regulation of colon cancer stem cells. Mol Cancer 2015; 14(98): 1-10.
[http://dx.doi.org/10.1186/s12943-015-0372-7] [PMID: 25928322]

[296] Zhang H, Mao F, Shen T, *et al.* Plasma miR-145, miR-20a, miR-21 and miR-223 as novel biomarkers for screening early-stage non-small cell lung cancer. Oncol Lett 2017; 13(2): 669-76.
[http://dx.doi.org/10.3892/ol.2016.5462] [PMID: 28356944]

[297] Yan LX, Huang XF, Shao Q, *et al.* MicroRNA miR-21 overexpression in human breast cancer is associated with advanced clinical stage, lymph node metastasis and patient poor prognosis. RNA 2008; 14(11): 2348-60.
[http://dx.doi.org/10.1261/rna.1034808] [PMID: 18812439]

[298] Wu H, Xiao Z, Wang K, Liu W, Hao Q. MiR-145 is downregulated in human ovarian cancer and modulates cell growth and invasion by targeting p70S6K1 and MUC1. Biochem Biophys Res Commun 2013; 441(4): 693-700.
[http://dx.doi.org/10.1016/j.bbrc.2013.10.053] [PMID: 24157791]

[299] Costa PM, Cardoso AL, Nóbrega C, *et al.* MicroRNA-21 silencing enhances the cytotoxic effect of the antiangiogenic drug sunitinib in glioblastoma. Hum Mol Genet 2013; 22(5): 904-18.
[http://dx.doi.org/10.1093/hmg/dds496] [PMID: 23201752]

[300] Qian C, Wang B, Zou Y, *et al.* MicroRNA 145 enhances chemosensivity of glioblastoma stem cells to demethoxycurcumin. Cancer Manag Res 2019; 11: 6829-40.
[http://dx.doi.org/10.2147/CMAR.S210076] [PMID: 31440081]

[301] Misso G, Di Martino MT, De Rosa G, *et al.* Mir-34: A new weapon against cancer? Mol Ther Nucleic Acids 2014; 3(9): e194-209.
[http://dx.doi.org/10.1038/mtna.2014.47] [PMID: 25247240]

[302] Liu C, Kelnar K, Liu B, *et al.* The microRNA miR-34a inhibits prostate cancer stem cells and metastasis by directly repressing CD44. Nat Med 2011; 17(2): 211-5.
[http://dx.doi.org/10.1038/nm.2284] [PMID: 21240262]

[303] Shi Y, Liu C, Liu X, Tang DG, Wang J. The microRNA miR-34a inhibits Non-Small Cell Lung Cancer (NSCLC) growth and the CD44hi stem-like NSCLC cells. PLoS One 2014; 9(3): e90022.
[http://dx.doi.org/10.1371/journal.pone.0090022] [PMID: 24595209]

[304]   Elmore S. Apoptosis: A review of programmed cell death. Toxicol Pathol 2007; 35(4): 495-516.
[http://dx.doi.org/10.1080/01926230701320337] [PMID: 17562483]

[305]   Jin Z, El-Deiry WS. Overview of cell death signaling pathways. Cancer Biol Ther 2005; 4(2): 139-63.
[http://dx.doi.org/10.4161/cbt.4.2.1508] [PMID: 15725726]

[306]   Thompson CB. Apoptosis in the pathogenesis and treatment of disease. Science 1995; 267(5203): 1456-62.
[http://dx.doi.org/10.1126/science.7878464] [PMID: 7878464]

[307]   Fulda S. How to target apoptosis signaling pathways for the treatment of pediatric cancers. Front Oncol 2013; 3(22): 22.
[http://dx.doi.org/10.3389/fonc.2013.00022] [PMID: 23420072]

[308]   Pfeffer CM, Singh ATK. Apoptosis: A target for anticancer therapy. Int J Mol Sci 2018; 19(2): 448-57.
[http://dx.doi.org/10.3390/ijms19020448] [PMID: 29393886]

[309]   Sayers TJ. Targeting the extrinsic apoptosis signaling pathway for cancer therapy. Cancer Immunol Immunother 2011; 60(8): 1173-80.
[http://dx.doi.org/10.1007/s00262-011-1008-4] [PMID: 21626033]

[310]   Wajant H. Death receptors. Essays Biochem 2003; 39: 53-71.
[http://dx.doi.org/10.1042/bse0390053] [PMID: 14585074]

[311]   Jendrossek V. The intrinsic apoptosis pathways as a target in anticancer therapy. Curr Pharm Biotechnol 2012; 13(8): 1426-38.
[http://dx.doi.org/10.2174/138920112800784989] [PMID: 22423614]

[312]   Walczak H. Death receptor-ligand systems in cancer, cell death, and inflammation. Cold Spring Harb Perspect Biol 2013; 5(5): a008698.
[http://dx.doi.org/10.1101/cshperspect.a008698] [PMID: 23637280]

[313]   Esposti MD. The roles of Bid. Apoptosis 2002; 7(5): 433-40.
[http://dx.doi.org/10.1023/A:1020035124855] [PMID: 12207176]

[314]   Ashkenazi A. Targeting the extrinsic apoptosis pathway in cancer. Cytokine Growth Factor Rev 2008; 19(3-4): 325-31.
[http://dx.doi.org/10.1016/j.cytogfr.2008.04.001] [PMID: 18495520]

[315]   Yin S, Xu L, Bandyopadhyay S, Sethi S, Reddy KB. Cisplatin and TRAIL enhance breast cancer stem cell death. Int J Oncol 2011; 39(4): 891-8.
[http://dx.doi.org/10.3892/ijo.2011.1085] [PMID: 21687939]

[316]   Plasilova M, Zivny J, Jelinek J, et al. TRAIL (Apo2L) suppresses growth of primary human leukemia and myelodysplasia progenitors. Leukemia 2002; 16(1): 67-73.
[http://dx.doi.org/10.1038/sj.leu.2402338] [PMID: 11840265]

[317]   Unterkircher T, Cristofanon S, Vellanki SH, et al. Bortezomib primes glioblastoma, including glioblastoma stem cells, for TRAIL by increasing tBid stability and mitochondrial apoptosis. Clin Cancer Res 2011; 17(12): 4019-30.
[http://dx.doi.org/10.1158/1078-0432.CCR-11-0075] [PMID: 21525171]

[318]   Dutta J, Fan Y, Gupta N, Fan G, Gélinas C. Current insights into the regulation of programmed cell death by NF-kappaB. Oncogene 2006; 25(51): 6800-16.
[http://dx.doi.org/10.1038/sj.onc.1209938] [PMID: 17072329]

[319]   Baud V, Karin M. Is NF-kappaB a good target for cancer therapy? Hopes and pitfalls. Nat Rev Drug Discov 2009; 8(1): 33-40.
[http://dx.doi.org/10.1038/nrd2781] [PMID: 19116625]

[320]   Zhou J, Zhang H, Gu P, Bai J, Margolick JB, Zhang Y. NF-kappaB pathway inhibitors preferentially inhibit breast cancer stem-like cells. Breast Cancer Res Treat 2008; 111(3): 419-27.

[http://dx.doi.org/10.1007/s10549-007-9798-y] [PMID: 17965935]

[321]   Guzman ML, Swiderski CF, Howard DS, *et al.* Preferential induction of apoptosis for primary human leukemic stem cells. Proc Natl Acad Sci USA 2002; 99(25): 16220-5.
[http://dx.doi.org/10.1073/pnas.252462599] [PMID: 12451177]

[322]   He YC, Zhou FL, Shen Y, Liao DF, Cao D. Apoptotic death of cancer stem cells for cancer therapy. Int J Mol Sci 2014; 15(5): 8335-51.
[http://dx.doi.org/10.3390/ijms15058335] [PMID: 24823879]

[323]   Peitzsch C, Kurth I, Kunz-Schughart L, Baumann M, Dubrovska A. Discovery of the cancer stem cell related determinants of radioresistance. Radiother Oncol 2013; 108(3): 378-87.
[http://dx.doi.org/10.1016/j.radonc.2013.06.003] [PMID: 23830195]

[324]   Holčaková J, Nekulová M, Orzol P, Vojtěšek B. Mechanisms of drug resistance and cancer stem cells. Klin Onkol 2014; 27(Suppl. 1): S34-41.
[http://dx.doi.org/10.14735/amko20141S34] [PMID: 24945535]

[325]   Lenos KJ, Vermeulen L. Cancer stem cells don't waste their time cleaning-low proteasome activity, a marker for cancer stem cell function. Ann Transl Med 2016; 4(24): 519-26.
[http://dx.doi.org/10.21037/atm.2016.11.81] [PMID: 28149881]

[326]   Borah A, Raveendran S, Rochani A, Maekawa T, Kumar DS. Targeting self-renewal pathways in cancer stem cells: Clinical implications for cancer therapy. Oncogenesis 2015; 4(11): e177-87.
[http://dx.doi.org/10.1038/oncsis.2015.35] [PMID: 26619402]

[327]   Rosa R, D'Amato V, De Placido S, Bianco R. Approaches for targeting cancer stem cells drug resistance. Expert Opin Drug Discov 2016; 11(12): 1201-12.
[http://dx.doi.org/10.1080/17460441.2016.1243525] [PMID: 27700193]

[328]   Turdo A, Veschi V, Gaggianesi M, *et al.* Meeting the challenge of targeting cancer stem cells. Front Cell Dev Biol 2019; 7(16): 16.
[http://dx.doi.org/10.3389/fcell.2019.00016] [PMID: 30834247]

[329]   Chanmee T, Ontong P, Kimata K, Itano N. Key roles of hyaluronan and its CD44 receptor in the stemness and survival of cancer stem cells. Front Oncol 2015; 5(180): 180.
[http://dx.doi.org/10.3389/fonc.2015.00180] [PMID: 26322272]

[330]   Yoshida GJ, Saya H. Therapeutic strategies targeting cancer stem cells. Cancer Sci 2016; 107(1): 5-11.
[http://dx.doi.org/10.1111/cas.12817] [PMID: 26362755]

[331]   Annett S, Robson T. Targeting cancer stem cells in the clinic: Current status and perspectives. Pharmacol Ther 2018; 187: 13-30.
[http://dx.doi.org/10.1016/j.pharmthera.2018.02.001] [PMID: 29421575]

[332]   Orza A, Casciano D, Biris A. Nanomaterials for targeted drug delivery to cancer stem cells. Drug Metab Rev 2014; 46(2): 191-206.
[http://dx.doi.org/10.3109/03602532.2014.900566] [PMID: 24697156]

[333]   Tang DG. Understanding cancer stem cell heterogeneity and plasticity. Cell Res 2012; 22(3): 457-72.
[http://dx.doi.org/10.1038/cr.2012.13] [PMID: 22357481]

[334]   Shibata M, Hoque MO. Targeting cancer stem cells: A strategy for effective eradication of cancer. Cancers (Basel) 2019; 11(5): 732-49.
[http://dx.doi.org/10.3390/cancers11050732] [PMID: 31137841]

[335]   Iseghohi SO. Cancer stem cells may contribute to the difficulty in treating cancer. Genes Dis 2016; 3(1): 7-10.
[http://dx.doi.org/10.1016/j.gendis.2016.01.001] [PMID: 30258875]

[336]   Relation T, Dominici M, Horwitz EM. Concise review: An (Im)penetrable shield: How the tumor microenvironment protects cancer stem cells. Stem Cells 2017; 35(5): 1123-30.
[http://dx.doi.org/10.1002/stem.2596] [PMID: 28207184]

[337] Insan MB, Jaitak V. New approaches to target cancer stem cells: Current scenario. Mini Rev Med Chem 2014; 14(1): 20-34.
[http://dx.doi.org/10.2174/13895575113136660107] [PMID: 24195662]

[338] Würth R, Barbieri F, Florio T. New molecules and old drugs as emerging approaches to selectively target human glioblastoma cancer stem cells. BioMed Res Int 2014; 2014: 126586.
[http://dx.doi.org/10.1155/2014/126586] [PMID: 24527434]

[339] Khan IN, Al-Karim S, Bora RS, Chaudhary AG, Saini KS. Cancer stem cells: A challenging paradigm for designing targeted drug therapies. Drug Discov Today 2015; 20(10): 1205-16.
[http://dx.doi.org/10.1016/j.drudis.2015.06.013] [PMID: 26143148]

[340] Vinogradov S, Wei X. Cancer stem cells and drug resistance: The potential of nanomedicine. Nanomedicine (Lond) 2012; 7(4): 597-615.
[http://dx.doi.org/10.2217/nnm.12.22] [PMID: 22471722]

[341] Shapira A, Livney YD, Broxterman HJ, Assaraf YG. Nanomedicine for targeted cancer therapy: Towards the overcoming of drug resistance. Drug Resist Updat 2011; 14(3): 150-63.
[http://dx.doi.org/10.1016/j.drup.2011.01.003] [PMID: 21330184]

[342] Burke AR, Singh RN, Carroll DL, Torti FM, Torti SV. Targeting cancer stem cells with nanoparticle-enabled therapies. J Mol Biomark Diagn 2012; (Suppl. 8): 1-8.
[http://dx.doi.org/10.4172/2155-9929.S8-003] [PMID: 24383043]

[343] Yameen B, Choi WI, Vilos C, Swami A, Shi J, Farokhzad OC. Insight into nanoparticle cellular uptake and intracellular targeting. J Control Release 2014; 190: 485-99.
[http://dx.doi.org/10.1016/j.jconrel.2014.06.038] [PMID: 24984011]

[344] Gustafson HH, Holt-Casper D, Grainger DW, Ghandehari H. Nanoparticle uptake: The phagocyte problem. Nano Today 2015; 10(4): 487-510.
[http://dx.doi.org/10.1016/j.nantod.2015.06.006] [PMID: 26640510]

[345] Lu B, Huang X, Mo J, Zhao W. Drug delivery using nanoparticles for cancer stem-like cell targeting. Front Pharmacol 2016; 7(84): 84.
[http://dx.doi.org/10.3389/fphar.2016.00084] [PMID: 27148051]

[346] Siafaka PI, Üstündağ Okur N, Karavas E, Bikiaris DN. Surface modified multifunctional and stimuli responsive nanoparticles for drug targeting: current status and uses. Int J Mol Sci 2016; 17(9): 1440-79.
[http://dx.doi.org/10.3390/ijms17091440] [PMID: 27589733]

[347] Navya PN, Kaphle A, Srinivas SP, Bhargava SK, Rotello VM, Daima HK. Current trends and challenges in cancer management and therapy using designer nanomaterials. Nano Converg 2019; 6(1): 23.
[http://dx.doi.org/10.1186/s40580-019-0193-2] [PMID: 31304563]

[348] Andrews TE, Wang D, Harki DA. Cell surface markers of cancer stem cells: Diagnostic macromolecules and targets for drug delivery. Drug Deliv Transl Res 2013; 3(2): 121-42.
[http://dx.doi.org/10.1007/s13346-012-0075-1] [PMID: 25787981]

[349] Qiu L, Li H, Fu S, Chen X, Lu L. Surface markers of liver cancer stem cells and innovative targeted-therapy strategies for HCC. Oncol Lett 2018; 15(2): 2039-48.
[http://dx.doi.org/10.3892/ol.2017.7568] [PMID: 29434903]

[350] Pan Y, Ma S, Cao K, *et al.* Therapeutic approaches targeting cancer stem cells. J Cancer Res Ther 2018; 14(7): 1469-75.
[http://dx.doi.org/10.4103/jcrt.JCRT_976_17] [PMID: 30589025]

[351] Karsten U, Goletz S. What makes cancer stem cell markers different? Springerplus 2013; 2(1): 301.
[http://dx.doi.org/10.1186/2193-1801-2-301] [PMID: 23888272]

[352] O'Donnell EA, Ernst DN, Hingorani R. Multiparameter flow cytometry: Advances in high resolution

analysis. Immune Netw 2013; 13(2): 43-54.
[http://dx.doi.org/10.4110/in.2013.13.2.43] [PMID: 23700394]

[353]   Greve B, Kelsch R, Spaniol K, Eich HT, Götte M. Flow cytometry in cancer stem cell analysis and separation. Cytometry A 2012; 81(4): 284-93.
[http://dx.doi.org/10.1002/cyto.a.22022] [PMID: 22311742]

[354]   Matsui WH. Cancer stem cell signaling pathways. Medicine (Baltimore) 2016; 95(1)(Suppl. 1): S8-S19.
[http://dx.doi.org/10.1097/MD.0000000000004765] [PMID: 27611937]

[355]   Wang J, Sullenger BA, Rich JN. Notch signaling in cancer stem cells. Adv Exp Med Biol 2012; 727: 174-85.
[http://dx.doi.org/10.1007/978-1-4614-0899-4_13] [PMID: 22399347]

[356]   Saygin C, Matei D, Majeti R, Reizes O, Lathia JD. Targeting cancer stemness in the clinic: From hype to hope. Cell Stem Cell 2019; 24(1): 25-40.
[http://dx.doi.org/10.1016/j.stem.2018.11.017] [PMID: 30595497]

[357]   Schreck KC, Taylor P, Marchionni L, *et al.* The Notch target Hes1 directly modulates Gli1 expression and Hedgehog signaling: A potential mechanism of therapeutic resistance. Clin Cancer Res 2010; 16(24): 6060-70.
[http://dx.doi.org/10.1158/1078-0432.CCR-10-1624] [PMID: 21169257]

[358]   Lau EY, Ho NP, Lee TK. Cancer stem cells and their microenvironment: Biology and therapeutic implications. Stem Cells Int 2017; 2017: 3714190.
[http://dx.doi.org/10.1155/2017/3714190] [PMID: 28337221]

[359]   Gattazzo F, Urciuolo A, Bonaldo P. Extracellular matrix: A dynamic microenvironment for stem cell niche. Biochim Biophys Acta 2014; 1840(8): 2506-19.
[http://dx.doi.org/10.1016/j.bbagen.2014.01.010] [PMID: 24418517]

[360]   Prieto-Vila M, Takahashi RU, Usuba W, Kohama I, Ochiya T. Drug resistance driven by cancer stem cells and their niche. Int J Mol Sci 2017; 18(12): 2574-95.
[http://dx.doi.org/10.3390/ijms18122574] [PMID: 29194401]

[361]   Zhang X, Nie D, Chakrabarty S. Growth factors in tumor microenvironment. Front Biosci 2010; 15: 151-65.
[http://dx.doi.org/10.2741/3612] [PMID: 20036812]

[362]   Imtiyaz HZ, Simon MC. Hypoxia-inducible factors as essential regulators of inflammation. Curr Top Microbiol Immunol 2010; 345: 105-20.
[http://dx.doi.org/10.1007/82_2010_74] [PMID: 20517715]

[363]   Turner MD, Nedjai B, Hurst T, Pennington DJ. Cytokines and chemokines: At the crossroads of cell signalling and inflammatory disease. Biochim Biophys Acta 2014; 1843(11): 2563-82.
[http://dx.doi.org/10.1016/j.bbamcr.2014.05.014] [PMID: 24892271]

[364]   Zhang S, Yang X, Wang L, Zhang C. Interplay between inflammatory tumor microenvironment and cancer stem cells. Oncol Lett 2018; 16(1): 679-86.
[http://dx.doi.org/10.3892/ol.2018.8716] [PMID: 29963133]

[365]   Parajuli P, Anand R, Mandalaparty C, *et al.* Preferential expression of functional IL-17R in glioma stem cells: Potential role in self-renewal. Oncotarget 2016; 7(5): 6121-35.
[http://dx.doi.org/10.18632/oncotarget.6847] [PMID: 26755664]

[366]   Ciardiello C, Leone A, Budillon A. The crosstalk between cancer stem cells and microenvironment is critical for solid tumor progression: The significant contribution of extracellular vesicles. Stem Cells Int 2018; 2018: 6392198.
[http://dx.doi.org/10.1155/2018/6392198] [PMID: 30532788]

[367]   Prahallad A, Bernards R. Opportunities and challenges provided by crosstalk between signalling pathways in cancer. Oncogene 2016; 35(9): 1073-9.

[http://dx.doi.org/10.1038/onc.2015.151] [PMID: 25982281]

[368] Begicevic RR, Falasca M. ABC transporters in cancer stem cells: Beyond chemoresistance. Int J Mol Sci 2017; 18(11): 2362-84.
[http://dx.doi.org/10.3390/ijms18112362] [PMID: 29117122]

[369] Choi CH. ABC transporters as multidrug resistance mechanisms and the development of chemosensitizers for their reversal. Cancer Cell Int 2005; 5(30): 30.
[http://dx.doi.org/10.1186/1475-2867-5-30] [PMID: 16202168]

[370] Dean M. ABC transporters, drug resistance, and cancer stem cells. J Mammary Gland Biol Neoplasia 2009; 14(1): 3-9.
[http://dx.doi.org/10.1007/s10911-009-9109-9] [PMID: 19224345]

[371] Sukowati CH, Rosso N, Crocè LS, Tiribelli C. Hepatic cancer stem cells and drug resistance: Relevance in targeted therapies for hepatocellular carcinoma. World J Hepatol 2010; 2(3): 114-26.
[http://dx.doi.org/10.4254/wjh.v2.i3.114] [PMID: 21160982]

[372] Deeley RG, Westlake C, Cole SP. Transmembrane transport of endo- and xenobiotics by mammalian ATP-binding cassette multidrug resistance proteins. Physiol Rev 2006; 86(3): 849-99.
[http://dx.doi.org/10.1152/physrev.00035.2005] [PMID: 16816140]

[373] Daood M, Tsai C, Ahdab-Barmada M, Watchko JF. ABC transporter (P-gp/ABCB1, MRP1/ABCC1, BCRP/ABCG2) expression in the developing human CNS. Neuropediatrics 2008; 39(4): 211-8.
[http://dx.doi.org/10.1055/s-0028-1103272] [PMID: 19165709]

[374] Li W, Zhang H, Assaraf YG, et al. Overcoming ABC transporter-mediated multidrug resistance: Molecular mechanisms and novel therapeutic drug strategies. Drug Resist Updat 2016; 27: 14-29.
[http://dx.doi.org/10.1016/j.drup.2016.05.001] [PMID: 27449595]

[375] Vaz AP, Ponnusamy MP, Batra SK. Cancer stem cells and therapeutic targets: An emerging field for cancer treatment. Drug Deliv Transl Res 2013; 3(2): 113-20.
[http://dx.doi.org/10.1007/s13346-012-0095-x] [PMID: 24077517]

[376] Relling MV. Are the major effects of P-glycoprotein modulators due to altered pharmacokinetics of anticancer drugs? Ther Drug Monit 1996; 18(4): 350-6.
[http://dx.doi.org/10.1097/00007691-199608000-00006] [PMID: 8857549]

[377] Wu C, Alman BA. Side population cells in human cancers. Cancer Lett 2008; 268(1): 1-9.
[http://dx.doi.org/10.1016/j.canlet.2008.03.048] [PMID: 18487012]

[378] Szakács G, Annereau JP, Lababidi S, et al. Predicting drug sensitivity and resistance: Profiling ABC transporter genes in cancer cells. Cancer Cell 2004; 6(2): 129-37.
[http://dx.doi.org/10.1016/j.ccr.2004.06.026] [PMID: 15324696]

[379] Liu C, Tang DG. MicroRNA regulation of cancer stem cells. Cancer Res 2011; 71(18): 5950-4.
[http://dx.doi.org/10.1158/0008-5472.CAN-11-1035] [PMID: 21917736]

[380] Khan AQ, Ahmed EI, Elareer NR, Junejo K, Steinhoff M, Uddin S. Role of miRNA-regulated cancer stem cells in the pathogenesis of human malignancies. Cells 2019; 8(8): 840-74.
[http://dx.doi.org/10.3390/cells8080840] [PMID: 31530793]

[381] Fan T, Wang W, Zhang B, et al. Regulatory mechanisms of microRNAs in lung cancer stem cells. Springerplus 2016; 5(1): 1762-72.
[http://dx.doi.org/10.1186/s40064-016-3425-5] [PMID: 27795904]

[382] Hao J, Zhang Y, Deng M, et al. MicroRNA control of epithelial-mesenchymal transition in cancer stem cells. Int J Cancer 2014; 135(5): 1019-27.
[http://dx.doi.org/10.1002/ijc.28761] [PMID: 24500893]

[383] Yeung KT, Yang J. Epithelial-mesenchymal transition in tumor metastasis. Mol Oncol 2017; 11(1): 28-39.
[http://dx.doi.org/10.1002/1878-0261.12017] [PMID: 28085222]

[384] Lamouille S, Xu J, Derynck R. Molecular mechanisms of epithelial-mesenchymal transition. Nat Rev Mol Cell Biol 2014; 15(3): 178-96.
[http://dx.doi.org/10.1038/nrm3758] [PMID: 24556840]

[385] Mittal V. Epithelial mesenchymal transition in tumor metastasis. Annu Rev Pathol 2018; 13: 395-412.
[http://dx.doi.org/10.1146/annurev-pathol-020117-043854] [PMID: 29414248]

[386] Herrera-Carrillo E, Liu YP, Berkhout B. Improving miRNA delivery by optimizing miRNA expression cassettes in diverse virus vectors. Hum Gene Ther Methods 2017; 28(4): 177-90.
[http://dx.doi.org/10.1089/hgtb.2017.036] [PMID: 28712309]

[387] Kota J, Chivukula RR, O'Donnell KA, *et al.* Therapeutic microRNA delivery suppresses tumorigenesis in a murine liver cancer model. Cell 2009; 137(6): 1005-17.
[http://dx.doi.org/10.1016/j.cell.2009.04.021] [PMID: 19524505]

[388] Shah MY, Ferrajoli A, Sood AK, Lopez-Berestein G, Calin GA. microRNA therapeutics in cancer - an emerging concept. EBioMedicine 2016; 12: 34-42.
[http://dx.doi.org/10.1016/j.ebiom.2016.09.017] [PMID: 27720213]

[389] Akbari Moqadam F, Pieters R, den Boer ML. The hunting of targets: Challenge in miRNA research. Leukemia 2013; 27(1): 16-23.
[http://dx.doi.org/10.1038/leu.2012.179] [PMID: 22836911]

[390] Hassan M, Watari H, AbuAlmaaty A, Ohba Y, Sakuragi N. Apoptosis and molecular targeting therapy in cancer. BioMed Res Int 2014; 2014: 150845.
[http://dx.doi.org/10.1155/2014/150845] [PMID: 25013758]

[391] Pistritto G, Trisciuoglio D, Ceci C, Garufi A, D'Orazi G. Apoptosis as anticancer mechanism: Function and dysfunction of its modulators and targeted therapeutic strategies. Aging (Albany NY) 2016; 8(4): 603-19.
[http://dx.doi.org/10.18632/aging.100934] [PMID: 27019364]

[392] Safa AR. Resistance to cell death and its modulation in cancer stem cells. Crit Rev Oncog 2016; 21(3-4): 203-19.
[http://dx.doi.org/10.1615/CritRevOncog.2016016976] [PMID: 27915972]

[393] Mohammad RM, Muqbil I, Lowe L, *et al.* Broad targeting of resistance to apoptosis in cancer. Semin Cancer Biol 2015; 35(Suppl.): S78-S103.
[http://dx.doi.org/10.1016/j.semcancer.2015.03.001] [PMID: 25936818]

[394] Zhang L, Tong X, Li J, *et al.* Apoptotic and autophagic pathways with relevant small-molecule compounds, in cancer stem cells. Cell Prolif 2015; 48(4): 385-97.
[http://dx.doi.org/10.1111/cpr.12191] [PMID: 26013704]

[395] Xu Y, So C, Lam HM, Fung MC, Tsang SY. Apoptosis reversal promotes cancer stem cell-like cell formation. Neoplasia 2018; 20(3): 295-303.
[http://dx.doi.org/10.1016/j.neo.2018.01.005] [PMID: 29476980]

[396] Kharkar PS. Cancer Stem Cell (CSC) inhibitors: A review of recent patents (2012-2015). Expert Opin Ther Pat 2017; 27(7): 753-61.
[http://dx.doi.org/10.1080/13543776.2017.1325465] [PMID: 28460551]

[397] Hu Q, Sun W, Wang C, Gu Z. Recent advances of cocktail chemotherapy by combination drug delivery systems. Adv Drug Deliv Rev 2016; 98: 19-34.
[http://dx.doi.org/10.1016/j.addr.2015.10.022] [PMID: 26546751]

[398] Chen LS, Wang AX, Dong B, Pu KF, Yuan LH, Zhu YM. A new prospect in cancer therapy: Targeting cancer stem cells to eradicate cancer. Chin J Cancer 2012; 31(12): 564-72.
[http://dx.doi.org/10.5732/cjc.011.10444] [PMID: 22507219]

[399] Enciu AM, Codrici ED, Popescu I, Mihai S, Albulescu R, Pistol Tanase C. Patents in cancer stem cells. Recent Pat Biomark 2015; 5(1): 3-13.

[400] Wu W. Patents related to cancer stem cell research. Recent Pat DNA Gene Seq 2010; 4(1): 40-5.
[http://dx.doi.org/10.2174/187221510790410840] [PMID: 20218958]

[401] Benitah SA, Angulo GP, Martin AC, Martin MP. Targeting metastasis stem cells through a fatty acid receptor (CD36). US20190106503, 2019.

[402] Hoque MO, Sidransky D, Oki A. Pharmaceutical agents targeting cancer stem cells. US20190091202, 2019.

[403] Jabbari E. Drug delivery system and method for targeting cancer stem cells. US20190054034, 2019.

[404] Shi Y. Targeting glioblastoma stem cells through the TLX-TET3 axis. US20190032055, 2019.

[405] Kosai K, Wang Y. Viral vector targeting cancer stem cells. US20180346929, 2018.

[406] Magnani JL. Antibodies for targeting cancer stem cells and treating aggressive cancers. US20180318325, 2018.

[407] Yang M, Liu D. Nanoparticle composition for use in targeting cancer stem cells and method for treatment of cancer. US20180193485, 2018.

[408] Utku N, Gullans SR. Etoposide and prodrugs thereof for use in targeting cancer stem cells. US20180042952, 2018.

[409] Xing J, Jiang Z. Application of omeprazole in preparation of liver cancer stem cell inhibitor. CN108685919, 2018.

[410] Li JC, David L, Li Y, Li W. New compound and composition for targeting cancer stem cell. CN107721958, 2018.

[411] Udugamasooriya GD, Raymond A, Minna J. Compositions and methods of targeting cancer stem cells. WO2018053472, 2018.

[412] Cheresh D, Wettersten H. Compositions and methods for targeting and killing alpha-v beta-3-positive cancer stem cells (CSCs) and treating drug resistant cancers. WO2018183894, 2018.

[413] Li JC, Jiang Z, Harry R, Li Y, Liu J, Li W. Novel group of STAT3 pathway inhibitors and cancer stem cell pathway inhibitors. JP2018076349, 2018.

[414] Yun OC, Oh JE. Gene expression system for targeting cancer stem cell and cancer cell. KR20180044141, 2018.

Author Index

SUBJECT INDEX

U

V

W

X

www.ingramcontent.com/pod-product-compliance
Lightning Source LLC
Chambersburg PA
CBHW041705210326
41598CB00007B/542